The
Metabolism Miracle

The
Metabolism
Miracle

3 EASY STEPS TO REGAIN CONTROL OF YOUR WEIGHT . . . PERMANENTLY

Diane Kress, RD, CDE

RODALE.

Exclusive direct mail edition published by Rodale Inc. in September 2011 with arrangement of Da Capo Press, a member of the Perseus Books Group.

Printed in the United States of America

Rodale Inc. makes every effort to use acid-free ♾, recycled paper ♻.

Interior before and after photographs were supplied by individuals participating in the Metabolism Miracle program.

Back cover photographs © Beth Bartell.

Book design by Christima Gaugler

Library of Congress Cataloging-in-Publication Data is on file with the publisher

ISBN: 978-1-60961-059-3

2 4 6 8 10 9 7 5 3 1   hardcover

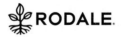

We inspire and enable people to improve their lives and the world around them.

For more of our products visit **rodalestore.com** or call 800-848-4735

*This book is dedicated with love and gratitude
to JC and Therese*

CONTENTS

PART FOUR
Recipes

A Plan for Your Body

In over twenty-five years, working with thousands of patients, I've met countless frustrated dieters. They walk through my office door, sit down across the desk from me, and describe their unsuccessful efforts to lose weight and keep it off. They often tell me that my office will be their last stop: "If this program doesn't work, I am giving up."

Diet after diet, pounds lost, pounds regained, they keep trying, they keep hoping, and yet they never get lasting results.

That all changes when they walk through my office door. By choosing this book, you've walked through the same door.

Diets are built on the assumption that everyone's metabolism works in the same way and that the diet that works for one person will work equally well for another. In other words, metabolism is metabolism and one size fits all. But what if your metabolism doesn't quite match the textbook version? What if your body works a little differently than the standard? What if you weren't failing at dieting, but your diet was failing you?

In fact, over 50 percent of patients seen in my practice for weight loss and weight-related health issues, as well as millions of people across the country and worldwide, really do have a very different metabolism than the type described as "normal." These people have tried diet after diet, having faithfully followed the rules that have produced results for their friends. Unbeknownst to them, those weight-loss programs can never work because they don't match the metabolism of these individuals.

If you find it impossible to lose weight and keep it off, even when you follow all the rules, there's an excellent chance that your metabolism doesn't match the cookie-cutter kind. The Metabolism Miracle was designed for people like you, to help you understand your body and learn to work with it rather than against it.

The Metabolism Miracle is not just another diet book. The program is the result of twenty-five years of working with thousands of patients whose metabolism did not follow the expected norm. Before I discovered the way to fuel this metabolism properly, they had little to no chance of permanent weight loss, no matter how hard they tried. Now they walk out my door with the potential for 100 percent success.

BE PREPARED TO BE SURPRISED

On any given day, over 35 percent of Americans—more than 71 million people—actively try to lose weight. As a result, the weight-loss industry has exploded with gimmicks and fads all promising a "slimmer, sexier, healthier you."

Yet as you look around, you will see more overweight people than ever before. More than 60 percent of the population is classified as overweight, and the numbers are escalating. Americans spend billions of dollars annually in the pursuit of quick, easy, and lasting weight loss. Ironically, as we spend more time, energy, and money than ever to lose weight, our population is heavier than ever before.

We are becoming sicker as a consequence. Many serious conditions are linked directly to weight. The risks of type 2 diabetes, cardiovascular disease, cancer, hypertension, acid reflux disease, sleep apnea, depression, and even infertility all increase as weight increases.

The long-term success rate of any of the available diet plans is a meager 2 percent. That means only two out of one hundred serious dieters have been able to maintain their weight loss at the end of five years. Ninety percent of dieters who have managed to lose weight regain all of it within one year! As a result, people jump from diet to diet, hoping to find the magic formula that will help them to lose unhealthy weight and keep it off for a lifetime. They spend years of their lives counting calories, spending "points," weighing and measuring food as well as their bodies, checking fat grams, checking sugar grams, and ultimately punishing themselves for falling off their program.

The Metabolism Miracle breaks through this dieting madness. For years, medical science recognized a one-size-fits-all metabolism, and standard diet programs were designed accordingly. More recently, researchers identified an alternative metabolism and categorized it under a variety of terms, including *metabolic syndrome, syndrome X*, and *insulin resistance*. Millions of people have this alternative metabolism, which I refer to as *Metabolism B*. Unfortunately, a diet has never been fully developed to work in tandem with all the special requirements of this type of metabolism. Up until now, there was no diet to rely upon for permanent weight loss.

If you have Metabolism B, you were born with a different blueprint for processing food. You may not always have had problems keeping weight off, but at some point over the years, the progressive nature of Metabolism B advanced to the point that you noticed the symptoms: progressive weight gain around the middle, fatigue, and carb cravings. Unchecked, the symptoms lead to health issues involving cholesterol, blood sugar, and blood pressure. Your body no longer abides by the dieting rules that work for others. Instead, you require a program that has been designed with your blueprint in mind.

The Metabolism Miracle program is a three-step approach that resists your body's overactive response to carbohydrate, trains your body to handle carbohydrate normally, and then teaches you to live a life in harmony with your unique metabolism. Once you learn to live in balance with your metabolism, your weight will come off and *permanently* stay off. Your health will improve, your energy level will soar, and you'll experience a feeling of peace and contentment. Miraculously, you will begin to feel the effects of this new approach in less than one week.

To determine if you have Metabolism B, you will complete a basic checklist that pinpoints the telltale signs, symptoms, and personal medical history that characterize people with Metabolism B. If you would like more in-depth proof, your most recent lab data can verify the results. Either way, your search for the right weight-loss program has ended.

The Metabolism Miracle will help you to understand the way your body works and empower you to work with your metabolism instead of against it. The Miracle will bring back the healthy you—no more carb cravings, energy slumps, food binges, or frustrating weight regain. You will learn about the foods that you can eat whenever you are hungry, with no calorie counting, weighing, or measuring. You'll also learn about the energy foods that will fuel your metabolism all day long. Weight-related health problems will diminish and even disappear. And you will feel healthier and more energized than you have felt in years or perhaps in your lifetime.

The Metabolism Miracle is easy, effective, and, best of all, the first and only program written expressly for *you*.

PART ONE

Your Metabolism Is Different

A PROGRAM TO CHANGE YOUR LIFE

You know who you are.

You have suffered through liquid diets, portion-controlled diets, calorie-counting diets, point diets, fat-free diets, carb-free diets, grapefruit diets, and doctor diets, only to regain every pound you lost. You sit at weight-loss support meetings next to people who succeed while you do not. You are an expert in dieting. You can recite the calorie content of foods without glancing at a book. You have tried, over and over. *You really have tried.*

Yet you have known for a long time that something is very different about your body. Others eat twice the quantity of food that you consume, yet they weigh much less than you. No matter what the doctors and nutritionists say, you insist that you must have a different metabolism.

You are right.

I know this because, like you, I have this different metabolism, and it confounded me for much of my life. *The Metabolism Miracle* is the culmination of my life's work in treating people with stubborn weight and weight-related maladies. But the story begins with my own body. I have spent more than twenty-five years as a registered dietitian specializing in weight loss, prevention and management of diabetes, and cardiovascular nutrition. Only after my own health declined and I pieced together clues from years of personal trial and error, the experience of thousands of patients, and current medical research did I finally find the answer.

The Metabolism Miracle changed my life and continues to keep my patients and me healthier than ever before.

A PERSONAL STORY

As a registered dietitian, trained in the traditional approach to nutrition, I have counseled thousands of people over the years and worked equally hard with all of them. Yet early in my clinical practice, I noticed something that deeply concerned me. More than 45 percent of those I counseled never achieved their desired results.

In the traditional school of thought, a person will gain weight if he or she consumes more calories than are burned off. Most weight-loss diets are based on this "law of calories." The fewer calories a person consumes, the less he or she will weigh. Add physical activity to the equation and weight loss accelerates. But the law of calories didn't apply to all of my patients.

For years, I used a universal formula for all of my weight-loss clients to determine the number of calories they should consume to lose weight. I dutifully plugged each patient's gender, height, desired weight, age, and physical activity into the formula and came up with a calorie allotment that should have guaranteed weight loss. If the patient's cholesterol was elevated, I added a saturated fat and dietary cholesterol restriction. If he or she suffered from hypertension, I added a sodium restriction. The formula then configured a nice, neat diet package with precise calorie allotments.

The patients followed the diet, weighed and measured food portions, kept detailed food journals, and exercised regularly. But many of them returned for their follow-up visits disillusioned and depressed.

Nothing significant had happened! They had lost little weight and had no real change in their blood lipids, blood sugar, or blood pressure. They remained on medications, and, worse yet, their medications increased over the years.

I sympathized, but I also wondered if they had truly followed my instructions. Perhaps they wrote what they believed I wanted to see in their food logs. Maybe, in reality, they didn't follow the plan or exercise. Perhaps they were overeating or sneaking in snacks. The diet worked for half of my clients, so why didn't it work for all of them?

As time passed, I realized that if I were to help these patients, I would have to challenge some of the principles that were written in stone by the medical community. There had to be a reason for the obesity epidemic. Why was type 2 diabetes afflicting more and younger people? Why were so few people succeeding at diets despite the billion-dollar weight-loss industry? Why were we becoming a nation reliant on prescription medications? Something had to be very wrong with the theories.

Then something alarming happened to me.

As a nutrition counselor with a thriving practice, I knew everything there was to know about diets; I could configure them in my sleep. I prided myself in following a balanced, healthful diet. I exercised regularly and practiced what I preached. But as I entered my thirties, my body changed.

At a routine physical exam, a nurse told me that my consistently low blood pressure had increased to the normal zone. Shortly after, my cholesterol and triglyceride levels began to rise, regardless of exercise and a low-fat, low-cholesterol lifestyle. Soon, even as I counted every calorie that passed my lips, the numbers on the scale began to creep upward. Worse yet, I noticed a small roll of fat around my middle!

I followed the guidelines that I had been taught were the key to good health. Like my patients, I monitored my calories, fat, cholesterol, and sodium, and I exercised faithfully. Despite all of this effort, I continued to gain weight and eventually needed medication to help control my blood pressure and cholesterol.

Finally, just before my fortieth birthday, I developed type 2 diabetes. What had happened? Nothing I did would stop this train! Despite my attempts to do everything by the book, my body would not respond. I finally felt the full force of the frustration and emotional pain that my patients endured.

The experience led me right back to the traditional nutrition theories that I had been teaching my patients. This time, I dug into the research, analyzed the nutrition "wisdom," and looked at the patterns that fit my successful patients and unsuccessful patients. I tested out new approaches, threw out those that didn't work, and came up with confirmation of what I had come to suspect: It was clear that one segment of dieters responded to the traditional approach. The other needed a very different and new approach. The Metabolism Miracle is that approach.

It worked. Within the first few weeks on the program, I felt like a new person, with higher energy, looser jeans, and no cravings. Within the second month, my doctor eliminated my hypertension medication and decreased my medication for cholesterol. Eventually, I no longer needed any of my medications, and my blood pressure, cholesterol, weight, and diabetes remained under good control! I felt great, and friends told me I looked ten years younger.

Not only did the program work for me, it worked for each patient who followed it. I erased the board of all the ideals I had once held as dietary gospel and I rewrote the diet book.

A DIFFERENT KIND OF METABOLISM

Most weight-loss advice recognizes only one metabolism, the version every medical student and dietetics student is currently taught. I call this *Metabolism A*. But as I failed to lose weight on standard diets written for Metabolism A, and as I watched many of my patients fail to lose weight on those diets, it became clear that we were working with a different animal, a metabolism that I refer to as *Metabolism B*. This alternative metabolism requires an entirely different approach, and that is how the Metabolism Miracle began to take shape.

You may be familiar with the labels *metabolic syndrome* and *insulin resistance*, terms designed by the medical community to recognize alternative metabolism. Together with a host of other signs that may seem unrelated, including fatigue, sleeplessness, mild depression, and anxiety, these conditions point to Metabolism B. Although alternative metabolism has been recognized for years, no diet to date addresses all the facets that contribute to this metabolism. As a result, all diets designed to match alternative metabolism have fallen short. The Metabolism Miracle takes the whole package of symptoms into account, stops the weight-gain train in its tracks, and even helps to reverse some of the health consequences of this metabolism.

Individuals with Metabolism B will never succeed at following a traditional weight-loss diet because their alternative metabolism follows a different set of rules than those of the standard metabolism. In fact, attempting to lose weight using a traditional approach can set off the downward spiral of unchecked Metabolism B.

The split between dieters with Metabolism A and Metabolism B is almost even. More than 45 percent of those struggling to lose weight were born with the genetic predisposition to Metabolism B. The onset of their symptoms is slow and progressive and may be expedited by a number of life events, including stress, weight gain, illness, and hormonal changes.

Take heart. You do not lack willpower! You are not a lazy dieter! You have not imagined impossible obstacles! Your body simply responds differently. Once you understand your body, you can work with your unique metabolism instead of against it. By identifying the category you were born into, you can easily make the right food choices to lead a healthy life at your healthy weight.

Because other diets haven't worked for people with Metabolism B, permanent weight loss can feel overwhelmingly difficult and often downright impossible. Add a health issue such as type 2 diabetes to the scenario and the extra weight becomes downright scary. I know because I've been there.

If you have the genes that have set you up for a lifetime of struggles with weight, the Metabolism Miracle will absolutely work for you. Before the Metabolism Miracle, you had little to no chance of permanent weight loss. With the program, you will reach and maintain a healthy weight, your lab data will improve, the dose of medications that you take to control weight-related health problems will decrease or disappear, and you may avoid health risks down the line.

Best of all, you will look and feel great!

2

IS THIS YOU?

Anyone can lose weight with the Metabolism Miracle, but the program is designed specifically for people who have Metabolism B and therefore have no chance of long-term weight-loss success with any other diet plan. They will, for the first time, lose weight and *successfully* keep it off for the rest of their lives because this approach, unlike other weight-loss programs, matches their unique metabolism.

You may be saying, "I must not have Metabolism B, because only two years ago I could control my weight with no problem." Keep in mind that people with Metabolism B have always had the genetic predisposition for this alternative metabolism, but it is only when an outside trigger, such as stress, weight, inactivity, or illness, flips the switch that Metabolism B begins to manifest itself in such symptoms as weight gain or high cholesterol. Some people show symptoms as children, and others show symptoms during the teen or adult years. The longer a person has been living with unchecked Metabolism B in its switched-on mode, the more progressive his or her weight gain and weight-related health issues become. (See "Trouble Triggers," page 28.)

How do you know if you have this alternate metabolism? When a patient walks into my office, often on a referral from a medical doctor, I listen to that person's weight-loss history and get a sense of his or her overall health, energy, and well-being. I review the family medical history and, if the patient has a blood profile from a recent visit to the doctor, I screen those numbers. All of these clues help me to identify whether the patient has Metabolism A or B. This chapter will help you to do the same.

To start, answer the following twelve descriptive questions. Most people with Metabolism B see themselves as they answer yes to questions on the list. If you recognize yourself in a number of them, you may have Metabolism B, and you should move on to the easy checklists that follow.

A LOOK IN THE MIRROR

_____ Have you dieted for years, perhaps successfully in the past, but now even tried-and-true diets you once relied upon for weight loss fail you?

_____ Do you notice that you can stick to a diet for only a short time, and you get so discouraged by the dismal results, constant hunger, and overwhelming cravings that you abandon your good intentions?

_____ Are you gaining weight regardless of your efforts, and is this weight shifting into a roll around your middle?

_____ Does the fat around your midsection look and feel spongy, loose, and watery?

_____ Can people around you eat more and yet weigh less than you?

_____ Is your overall health—physical, mental, and emotional—declining as your weight increases?

_____ Do you need medical prescriptions for weight-related health problems such as hypertension, cholesterol, triglycerides, acid reflux, insomnia, depression, anxiety, or arthritis pain?

_____ Despite diet and exercise, has your doctor been forced to increase your medication dosages or add new prescriptions to maintain your health?

_____ Do cravings sometimes gnaw at you like an addiction, and do you feel a strong urge to eat carbohydrates such as candy, sweets, bread, pasta, or chips?

_____ Do you feel depressed, irritable, unattractive, and undesirable?

_____ Are you fatigued, even after a proper amount of sleep?

_____ Do you miss the "old you"?

If you found yourself answering yes to several of these questions, go directly to the following simple checklist of symptoms to learn whether the

Metabolism Miracle can help you regain your health and sense of well-being and lose weight forever. If you answer no to all of these checkpoints, it's quite possible that you have textbook metabolism, Metabolism A, and can lose weight on any good weight-loss program.

CLUES TO METABOLISM B

This list of symptoms is one of the first pieces of information I use when trying to identify Metabolism A or Metabolism B. It still surprises me that when people with Metabolism A read the checklist, they identify with only a few of the symptoms, whereas people with Metabolism B relate to many, if not most, of them.

Check off any of the following experiences that describe a day in your life.

_____ You tire easily and frequently feel fatigued, even upon awakening.

_____ You feel mildly depressed.

_____ You feel an energy slump in the late afternoon.

_____ You frequently feel anxious.

_____ You crave carbohydrate foods, such as bread, chips, sweets, or pasta.

_____ Your midsection has a roll of fat.

_____ You gain weight easily and find it difficult to lose weight.

_____ You have trouble sleeping.

_____ You are often forgetful and worry about your short-term memory.

_____ You have racing thoughts.

_____ Your sexual drive has declined.

_____ You find it difficult to focus and concentrate and are easily distracted.

_____ Bright light or headlights at night bother you.

_____ You are irritable and have a "short fuse."

_____ You have increased sensitivity to aches and pains.

_____ Your eyes frequently tear up and at other times feel dry and irritated.

_____ You have frequent dull headaches.

_____ You feel slightly dizzy, flushed, or "weak in the knees" after even a little bit of alcohol.

If you have identified with twelve or more of the clues on this symptoms checklist, you likely have Metabolism B.

You may have looked at the symptoms checklist for Metabolism B and thought that they could be attributed to many different conditions, including menopause, chronic fatigue syndrome, midlife, or even a high-stress job. But at the end of eight weeks on Step One of the Metabolism Miracle, many symptoms from the checklist will disappear along with weight because the symptoms stem from untreated Metabolism B.

Any symptoms that persist are related to something else and should be addressed from another angle. For example, if after eight weeks a patient still has panic attacks, it would be prudent to discuss them with his or her physician.

Ann's Epiphany

When Ann first came to my Nutrition Center, she checked off many of the symptoms from the checklist. She smiled when she handed the list to me, saying, "Of course I feel this way. These symptoms are due to menopause and, honey, I'm there."

I agreed that the symptoms could relate to many conditions—menopause, fibromyalgia, chronic fatigue syndrome, and just plain aging. But once people begin the Metabolism Miracle program, they quickly discover whether their metabolism may be to blame for many of the unpleasant symptoms.

Ann started the three-step Metabolism Miracle program and, a few weeks later, she sent me an e-mail message with only two words: "It lifted." When she returned to the office after eight weeks, she was beaming. "I can't believe it! Almost all of the symptoms I attributed to menopause—my mild depression, periods of anxiety, poor sleep, midline fat, weight gain, fatigue, forgetfulness—are all so much better." Ann had lost inches of fat and was already wearing smaller-size slacks, but mostly she was thrilled to feel like her old self again.

Still, she couldn't understand why one symptom hadn't changed. "I am still irritable and have a short fuse." I had to laugh and explain that the program can't fix everything: "Ann, you are just plain irritable with a short fuse!"

BLAME IT ON THE GENES: 22 HEALTH CONDITIONS AFFECTED BY METABOLISM B

Certain medical conditions are very common in people with Metabolism B. They range from high cholesterol to type 2 diabetes. The longer you live your life without treating Metabolism B properly, the greater the chance that you will develop some of these medical problems. The sooner you start the Metabolism Miracle, the more likely you are to avoid these problems in the future or, as is often the case, the more likely you can reverse them.

Many of these conditions work in a domino-like chain effect, with the genetic profile for Metabolism B starting the reaction. For example, it is Metabolism B's excessive insulin release that causes midline fat to accumulate. That midline fat in turn provokes hypertension and acid reflux (GERD). In another chain, excess insulin in the bloodstream promotes excess circulating fats such as cholesterol and triglycerides, and they in turn contribute to heart disease. Fluctuating blood sugar levels, a direct result of unchecked Metabolism B, can contribute to mild depression, anxiety, panic attacks, and short-term memory loss. Hormonal imbalance can cause polycystic ovarian syndrome and irregularity in menstrual cycles and may even contribute to infertility. You get the picture.

If you are young and haven't experienced any of these conditions, don't wave them off. Look at your family's medical history and ascertain if parents, siblings, grandparents, aunts, or uncles have had any of the following medical conditions.

Almost all of the medical conditions listed at right require medication. When you fuel your metabolism correctly, with a measured carbohydrate dose in the strategically timed pattern designed in the Metabolism Miracle, the need for that medication may actually decline. You'll need less medication as you enjoy improved mental, physical, and emotional health; increased energy; and weight loss.

If you've experienced any of the following twenty-two medical conditions, you may want to read more about them and how they relate to your Metabolism B. For a detailed explanation of the following medical conditions, see the glossary.

22 HEALTH CONDITIONS THAT ARE AFFECTED BY METABOLISM B

_____ ADD or ADHD (attention deficit disorder or attention deficit/ hyperactivity disorder)

_____ Anxiety or panic attacks

_____ Cholesterol increases: total cholesterol, LDL ("bad") cholesterol, and/or triglycerides

_____ Low levels of HDL ("good") cholesterol

_____ Chronic fatigue

_____ Mild depression

_____ Prediabetes

_____ Type 2 diabetes

_____ Gestational diabetes (occurs only during pregnancy)

_____ Fibromyalgia

_____ GERD (gastroesophageal reflux disease)

_____ High blood pressure or recent increases in blood pressure

_____ Hypoglycemia (low blood sugar)

_____ Hypothyroidism (underactive thyroid—are you taking Synthroid or Levoxyl?)

_____ Infertility related to hormonal imbalance

_____ Metabolic syndrome

_____ Midline fat deposits (a roll around your middle) and increasing weight without increasing food intake

_____ Osteoarthritis

_____ Osteoporosis or osteopenia

_____ PCOS (polycystic ovarian syndrome; symptoms may include irregular menstrual period, heavy blood flow, clotting, severe PMS, and irregular endocrine reproductive hormonal patterns)

_____ Sleep apnea

_____ Sleep disturbances

If you have identified with twelve or more of the clues on the symptoms checklist on page 10, you likely have Metabolism B. If, in addition, you or a close relative currently has or has had several of the twenty-two medical conditions linked to Metabolism B, the case is even stronger for Metabolism B. Still skeptical? You may want to look at your most recent blood profile.

A PEEK AT YOUR NUMBERS

It is not necessary to have lab work done before beginning the Metabolism Miracle program. But if you have had blood work drawn within the past six months, compare your numbers to the Metabolism Miracle target range below. Keep in mind that the ranges used for this program are stricter than the American Medical Association's current recommendations because, not only does the Miracle help you to keep off weight, it also focuses on preventing medical problems in the future.

If you take medication to help control blood pressure, cholesterol, or blood sugar, your findings may appear in the normal range because they are being "Band-Aided." Ask yourself, "If I were not on medication, would these readings be normal?" Remember that this lab work needs to be drawn as *fasting* blood work (taken after at least eight hours without food or calorie-containing beverages).

Place a check on any line in which your numbers fall within the Metabolism B range.

	NORMAL	METABOLISM B
_____ *Fasting* blood glucose	65–99	90 or above
_____ Total cholesterol	Less than 200	200 or above
_____ LDL cholesterol	Less than 100	100 or above
_____ HDL cholesterol	Greater than 45	Less than 45
_____ Cholesterol/HDL ratio	Less than 5	Greater than 4
_____ Triglycerides	Less than 150	100 or above
_____ Hemoglobin A1C	Less than 6.0	Greater than 6.0
_____ Blood pressure	Less than 130/80	Greater than 130/80

If you checked off a fasting glucose of 90 or above, you have Metabolism B and can rest assured that the Metabolism Miracle will work for you. The more lab results that are out of range, the more influence Metabolism B has had on your health to this point. One of the goals of the Miracle is to get your lab work as close to normal as possible with as little medication as possible. In as little as eight weeks, your physician may need to lower your dosage of medication as your body enters a healthier zone.

For more information and background on how Metabolism B can lead to blood sugar conditions, please see chapter 12.

FINDING THE HIDDEN HEALTH CLUES

Before attempting any weight-loss program with my patients, I must first determine if they have Metabolism A or Metabolism B. Without this clarification, close to half of all dieters will not be able to lose weight permanently because most weight-loss programs do not match their alternative metabolism.

Each clue helps me to build the case for Metabolism B. But it's the whole picture that really tells the story.

Joanne: A Midlife Crisis?

Consider the case of forty-three-year-old Joanne, who is battling the midlife bulge. A mother of three children who range in age from five to sixteen, Joanne works part-time from her home office, exercises to stay physically fit, and vows to grow older "kicking and screaming."

She called my office in a panic. She explained that she can count calories in her sleep and can recite word for word the mantra of most diet programs. In the past, when her jeans felt snug, Joanne would join a popular diet program along with friends, all of whom seem to be battling weight at some level, and she was able to take off the excess weight in a reasonable amount of time.

Recently, things had changed for reasons that perplexed Joanne. She had been feeling mildly depressed and fatigued and—despite repeated attempts at weight loss, despite increasing her gym visits from three to five days per week, despite using the same diet program that she had always used to lose weight—she could not keep off the pounds. She had developed an annoying paunch, and no abdominal workout could budge it.

A self-confessed "carboholic," Joanne said that she was very strict with her eating and aggressive with her workouts. A doctor had once told her she had hypoglycemia, but she took no medication, and she couldn't understand why I wanted to see her lab work. She was tired, frustrated, angry with her body, and disgusted with what she saw in the mirror. After Joanne told me her story, completed the checklist of symptoms, and jotted down her weight and family medical histories, I had a sense of what she was up against. Her blood work confirmed it.

Joanne was not making mistakes with her diet or exercise plan. At some time over the past few years, Joanne's body began to show the progressive symptoms of Metabolism B. She no longer processed carbohydrate as she once did, and her weight had escalated.

Joanne began the Metabolism Miracle that day. She crossed her fingers as she left my office, and I told her that there was no need for luck this time. The program would work.

Eight weeks later, she returned for her first follow-up glowing, in new jeans and a form-fitting top. Her body had lost its excess layer of fat and the belly bulge was gone. She had energy, felt healthy, and looked great. Joanne continues to live the Metabolism Miracle lifestyle and maintains her desired weight!

That sounds fine, you say, for someone who has the luxury of dedicating so much time to her eating patterns and exercise regimen. But what about someone whose schedule makes flexibility impossible? What about someone who works full-time and travels frequently?

Joanne's Clues

- Midline fat
- Couldn't lose weight on her tried-and-true diets
- Decreased calories and increased physical activity but no weight loss
- Hypoglycemia
- Mother with prediabetes and a sister with gestational diabetes
- Craving for carbohydrates
- Fatigue and mild depression
- Short fuse and irritability

Michael: Changing the Future

Michael, a fifty-one-year-old traveling businessman, had just been diagnosed with type 2 diabetes when his assistant called my office, on a doctor's suggestion, to set up an appointment ASAP to "get this thing under control."

Michael arrived frazzled and distracted. His cell phone rang incessantly, and he kept checking his wristwatch as he curtly answered my questions. As we went through his history, Michael finally made eye contact and began to tell his story. Although his mother had tried hard and had listened to her physician's direction regarding her dietary intake and medications, she never had good control of her blood sugar. Michael had watched his beloved mother lose her vision and kidney function and eventually reside in a nursing home, totally dependent on others for her care and enduring kidney dialysis three days a week. She had recently died of complications from type 2 diabetes. Michael wiped his eyes several times as he told this story. "I don't want to end up like my mother," he said.

Michael worked long hours, traveled for business, ate many of his meals in restaurants, and wasn't Betty Crocker in the kitchen. He was divorced and lived alone. He was exhausted, frustrated, and annoyed with this diagnosis, and he felt he didn't have the time or energy to turn it around.

At five foot ten and 230 pounds, Michael did not exercise. Even with his medication for hypertension and cholesterol, his blood pressure was slightly elevated and his cholesterol/triglycerides exceeded the normal range. When the doctor handed Michael a prescription for oral medication for diabetes, he mentioned that the other medications would soon be increased. Michael hated the idea of more. He was disgusted with his expanding belly, and he disliked the person he had become—irritable, nasty, short-tempered, and so very tired.

A diagnosis of type 2 diabetes immediately identified Michael as having Metabolism B. But he had plenty of other clues as well. I asked Michael to keep an open mind and listen to what he needed to do to regain and maintain good health, peace of mind, and lots of energy. I explained the physiology of type 2 diabetes and how this program would, most likely, help to control his blood sugar without medication. I explained how the Metabolism Miracle would decrease the fat around his middle and the fat circulating in

Michael's Clues

- General overweight and lots of midline fat
- Elevated cholesterol/triglycerides
- Hypertension
- Type 2 diabetes
- Mother with type 2 diabetes
- Feeling anxious, frazzled, irritable
- Easily distracted
- Fatigue

his blood vessels, decrease his medications, and fit well into his chaotic lifestyle. He could still eat out, and there was no need for him to take cooking lessons!

Michael could adapt each step of the Metabolism Miracle diet to his lifestyle. We planned portable snacks, quick meals, and restaurant meals. For exercise, he would spend a half hour briskly walking back and forth to the train station.

After eight weeks of excellent blood sugar results without medication, a weight loss of ten pounds, and his physician already considering a decrease in his cholesterol medication, Michael saw a bright prognosis for long-term health and realized he would not have to live a difficult or complicated lifestyle.

It's been more than two years since that initial appointment, and Michael looks and feels great. He continues to follow the maintenance phase of the Miracle and, over the years, has referred many friends and clients to the Nutrition Center to "get their act together."

THIS IS YOU

You now know that your metabolism is different. You will no longer try to fit a square peg into a round hole, because the Metabolism Miracle is a lifetime lifestyle plan that is right for your metabolism. It will help you to lose weight, keep it off, and improve your emotional and physical well-being with as little medication as possible.

You may have been frustrated by weight gain for too long, your lab numbers may be abnormal, and you may have several serious health diagnoses, but that will all improve with the Miracle. Follow the program carefully and you will feel your body begin to change within a week. In as little as eight weeks, you will see major improvements in your weight as well as your physical, emotional, and mental health.

REAL READER SUCCESS STORY
Beth Bartell

Since August 2009, Beth has lost fifty-seven pounds.

Favorite MM Recipes: Miracle Quiche (page 219), Easy Egg Cups (page 218)

Beth, a middle school principle from Missouri, has battled with her weight since her two children were born. After the birth of her second child ten years ago, she found success on Weight Watchers—until she learned how to cheat on it and stopped seeing results.

On January 1, 2009, standing at five foot four and weighing 197 pounds, Beth once again vowed to lose weight. During dinner with friends a couple of weeks later, she listened as one woman talked about running the St. Louise half marathon that April. "It had to be the margaritas talking, but I agreed to join her! For twelve weeks, I miserably followed the 'calories in, calories out' approach to eating and exercising," Beth says. She dropped 20 pounds and finished the race, but an injury she received during the race pushed her off the wagon, and she was back up to 190 pounds by the end of the summer.

Beth discovered the Metabolism Miracle that August and hit her goal weight of 135 less than a year later, in May 2010. She is now on

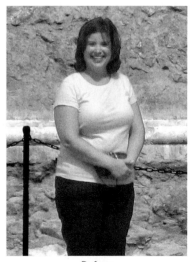

Before

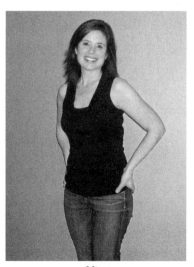

After

Step Three, the maintenance phase, and has stayed close to that number ever since. "Anytime I tried to lose weight in the past, I would obsess over the calories or the minutes exercising, and once I got bored with it, I gave up," she admits. "I didn't want to fail again, but MM was so easy to stick with."

Beth noticed that, unlike with other plans she had tried, she never hit a plateau on the Metabolism Miracle. In her "worst" month, she still lost 2 pounds. "I've never had that kind of luck on any other plan," she says.

Beth has noticed changes not only on the scale but in every aspect of her daily life: "While following MM, my energy abounds. I sleep like a champ and have never felt healthier! I'm no longer borderline diabetic, and I don't catch the bugs my kids bring home from school."

Although she praises the plan's user-friendliness, getting started took a few adjustments. "The hardest part was breakfast during Step One," she says, "just because I have to be at work so early, and I was never a breakfast person before starting the diet." Her shortcut to success was to make crustless quiches ahead of time and eat them for breakfast over the next few days. After Step One, she settled into a routine, eating a whole-grain English muffin with peanut butter and jelly every day for breakfast and a ham sandwich on whole-grain bread for lunch. With a husband and two kids, she needs to mix up dinner, but she can always find something for herself that fits into the plan. Thanks to MM food served at family mealtimes, Beth's twelve-year-old daughter has also trimmed down a bit, sidestepping a burgeoning weight problem.

What surprises Beth most is that she doesn't miss many of the foods she used to crave. "After starting the plan, I didn't even miss sweets anymore," she says. "I haven't had a french fry since I began the diet, and people are amazed." That doesn't stop her from finding diet-friendly ways to indulge, however: "Every night before I go to bed, I treat myself to some no-sugar added ice cream. I can get through the day if I know that's coming."

In April 2010, Beth ran the St. Louis half marathon again, shaving forty minutes off her time and finishing without injuries. Now, at her goal weight, she's training to do it again. "When it came to weight loss, I felt like a pretty big loser," she says, "but through MM, I've learned that I can do something and stick with it."

Beth's Advice

"Don't doubt yourself. Muscle through it those first few days, and it gets much easier."

3

UNDERSTANDING YOUR UNIQUE METABOLISM

I want to assure you that the Metabolism Miracle is not just another low-carb diet. Every other low-carb diet was written for the general public as a means to lose weight and, in some cases, decrease blood lipids. You can never achieve permanent weight loss on standard low-carb diets that haphazardly introduce the amount, type, and timing of carbohydrates. Standard low-carb diets used by those with metabolism B cause weight regain as soon as carbohydrate is reintroduced.

Unlike other low-carb diets, the three steps of the Metabolism Miracle program were designed to *retrain* your body to process carbohydrate normally rather than overreacting to it. Before you begin the program, it will help to understand how your metabolism differs and causes you to struggle with weight and related health conditions.

Think of your weight and any related health issues as the offshoots of a weed. If you simply treat the offshoots with diet restrictions and medications but don't get to the root, the weed will grow back, often even stronger.

Metabolism B causes your body to overreact to carbohydrate by releasing excess insulin, a fat-storage hormone. Too much insulin causes excess fat storage in both the blood (in the form of cholesterol and triglycerides) and the body (in the form of that roll of fat around your middle). The roots of your weight and medical problems include excess insulin release, resistance to your own insulin, and an overreaction to blood sugar. Once you destroy the root, the offshoots—weight, cholesterol, hypertension, and blood sugar issues—will wither away and stay under control with little to no medication.

Although other diets may succeed for a short period of time, they can't maintain weight loss, because they fail to work with your body's reaction to carbohydrate. *The Metabolism Miracle* is written to get to the root and retrain your body to process carbohydrate in a normal way.

Knowing exactly what is different about your body is half the battle. The other half is in learning how to treat this difference. That's where the Metabolism Miracle program comes in and empowers you to work with your body instead of against it.

A BAGEL IN THE LIFE OF METABOLISMS A AND B

To understand how Metabolism B reacts to carbohydrates, let's compare you with a friend who has Metabolism A.

You and your friend plan to spend the day shopping. On your way to the mall, you decide to stop for a bagel and coffee. A bagel contains carbohydrate, so as it digests, it turns into glucose that is released into the bloodstream. The brain detects this rise in blood glucose and instructs the pancreas to release the right amount of insulin to help bring the blood glucose back into the normal range. Glucose above the normal range will be used to refill glycogen stores in the muscle cells (the stores that you use to move, exercise, and even breathe) and fat cells (the stores that you burn when your muscle and liver stores have been depleted).

Think of insulin as the key that opens the cells' door to allow glucose to enter. Your friend's pancreas released just enough insulin to keep her blood glucose in the normal range, replenish the liver and the muscle cells, and store any excess in fat cells. After eating her bagel, your friend feels full and will remain satisfied during the four to five hours that this process takes.

Your pancreas, however, because of Metabolism B, releases excess insulin to deal with the bagel's glucose rush. Once this insulin helps to refill the glycogen stores in your muscle and liver, the excess keys will open excess fat cells. In an effort to feed these fat cells, you will dip into your normal blood sugar, leaving too little glucose in the bloodstream to keep up your energy and sense of satiation. Your blood glucose has now dipped below the normal range.

And so, after eating exactly the same meal, you will end up "fatter" than your friend and with lower blood glucose than she has! Your brain senses the low blood glucose, and you begin to feel tired, washed out, and hungry. This all happens only two hours after eating. You look at your friend—she feels great, with no fatigue or hunger. What a woman!

You feel the urge for a chocolate bar *now!* Your brain has caused you to crave carbohydrates, the one type of food that will quickly bring blood glucose up to normal. You start to feel a bit light-headed, empty, and irritable. Meanwhile, your friend shops away merrily.

If you cave in and eat that bar, you will immediately feel better, but only for a short time. The carbohydrates contained in the bar will return your blood glucose to normal, and, relieved, you will think to yourself, "This is the best chocolate bar on earth!" You accuse yourself of being a carboholic. But although you may appear to be out of control, gobbling carbs even as you desperately desire to lose weight, you are really a person following the direction of your brain to bring your blood glucose into a reasonable range.

The satisfaction lasts only a short time. When the chocolate bar digests and your blood sugar begins to rise, your brain once again calls upon your pancreas, and once again your pancreas, in its Metabolism B mode, releases too much insulin. The cycle has repeated itself, and excess fat cells receive the glucose while your blood glucose levels again dip. You are slowly becoming fatter, and, to add insult to injury, the insulin receptors on your fat cells are stretching, making it more difficult to open the cells (see "The Key to Insulin Resistance," page 25). Your energy level is dropping again, and you will soon need lunch.

You don't want to ask your friend to stop for lunch already. What if you simply ignore your brain and refuse to give in and eat? What if you remain steadfast and ignore your cravings? Will you be thinner if you ignore carb cravings? Surprisingly, the answer for people with Metabolism B is no.

THE BEAST WITHIN

The human body has a built-in survival mechanism that adds to the challenges of people with Metabolism B and thwarts the weight loss you hope to achieve as you skip a meal. When blood glucose drops to the low end of normal and you choose not to eat, your liver can feed the body.

The body has a five-hour clock that runs continually, day and night. Each time you eat carbohydrate, your body can run on that blood sugar for about five hours. If you choose not to eat within five hours, your liver will release stored blood glucose called *glycogen* that will push blood levels back into the normal range. Releases of liver glycogen keep your body working until you choose to eat again.

If you have ever gone to bed hungry and the next morning you wake up no longer hungry, you are feeling the effects of the self-feeding response.

The Key to Insulin Resistance

You know now that your plumped-up fat cells and weight gain come from the hyper-insulin release that characterizes Metabolism B. But people with Metabolism B have another challenge as well.

Imagine that insulin is a key that must fit perfectly into a keyhole to open a lock. If the keyhole is misshapen, the key can no longer fit. With Metabolism B, as fat cells grow in size, their keyholes change shape until the insulin keys can no longer fit to open the cell door, a condition called *insulin resistance*. Blood sugar remains in the bloodstream and, as a result, the pancreas works harder than ever to release more insulin that will fit the keyholes, all to no avail. You've eaten, but your cells aren't being "fed," and you end up feeling tired, depressed, fatigued, and very hungry.

A person with "normal" Metabolism A has keyholes that can never change, no matter how fat or how thin he or she becomes. Regardless of how large a Metabolism A person's fat cells become, insulin keys will always fit the insulin receptor keyholes and will always open the cell to receive the glucose. With Metabolism A, a 350-pound man's insulin will fit his insulin receptors as perfectly as it did when he weighed 200 pounds.

When insulin resistance is left untreated, the fatigued pancreas can no longer release enough insulin, and much of the insulin that it does release can't fit the keyholes. Continuously facing the locked doors, blood glucose backs up in the bloodstream. This is the beginning of type 2 diabetes and explains why it's so important to use the Metabolism Miracle to get this problem under control before it turns into an irreversible health challenge.

Similarly, if you work through lunch without eating, you might feel hungry for a little while, and then the hunger passes. Your liver took care of you by releasing glycogen to raise your blood glucose and satisfy the brain.

When you and your friend decided to postpone lunch, you both passed the five-hour mark and your livers released glycogen. But your friend with Metabolism A released the right amount of insulin, whereas your body over-released insulin and then ferried the liver's sugar from your bloodstream into your fat cells. You will actually gain weight because you did not eat within five hours!

As a result of that hyper-insulin response, you feel exhausted and irritable. You are developing a midline paunch, your blood pressure and cholesterol may be rising, and you may be crossing the boundary into the tricky waters of diabetes. You constantly struggle with bouts of low blood sugar that have turned you into a carbohydrate addict. No wonder your self-esteem has plummeted and you feel out of control!

It may not seem fair, but your overactive pancreas and resistance to insulin will increase your appetite, weight, and related health issues while wreaking havoc on your life. That is, until you learn to work with it rather than against it.

You haven't gained weight because you've eaten too much fat, sugar, or calories. You've gained weight because your body releases excess insulin, which opens excess fat cells. Those fat cells are fed at the expense of your normal blood sugar, and that depletes your energy level. Of course, you crave more food as a result! You haven't caused these problems, but you *can* improve and even correct them. The three steps of the Metabolism Miracle will help you to do it.

You may or may not have heard your doctor mention insulin resistance when assessing your blood glucose. Remember that the longer someone has lived with the switched-on Metabolism B, the more progressive that person's health problems become. Most people know that they weigh much more than they should, given what they eat, and that they can't lose weight and keep it off and that they feel awful and may be getting sicker. But they may not know they have insulin resistance, metabolic syndrome, and/or a host of other maladies that are related to their alternative metabolism. Insulin resistance is only one of many symptoms that characterize Metabolism B.

The Bagel Bomb

Depending upon your metabolism, a bagel can cause two very different reactions in the body. This chart illustrates how the paths diverge.

You and your friend both eat a bagel.

↓

The bagel's carbohydrate turns to blood glucose and enters the bloodstream.

↓

The brain senses the blood glucose rise and instructs the pancreas to release the hormone insulin.

METABOLISM A AND THE BAGEL

↓

The pancreas releases exactly the right amount of insulin to handle the rise in blood glucose.

↓

Insulin acts like a key and opens the right amount of fat and muscle cells and returns the glucose in the bloodstream to normal.

↓

Glucose from the bagel provides immediate energy and replaces glycogen in muscle and liver, and any excess is stored as fat.

↓

Equilibrium results in the body feeling satisfied and full after the meal.

↓

Satisfaction lasts for four to five hours, until hunger naturally occurs.

METABOLISM B (YOU) AND THE BAGEL

↓

The pancreas overreacts and releases excess insulin to handle the rise in blood glucose.

↓

Excess insulin opens excess fat cells, ushers in the glucose, and leaves too little glucose in the blood for basic energy. Your fat cells get microscopically larger and receptors "stretch" a bit.

↓

The brain signals you to eat more carbohydrate to quickly raise the blood glucose. You feel hungry, tired, shaky, nauseated, and irritable until you eat a carbohydrate snack.

↓

You temporarily feel better as blood glucose rises.

↓

Your brain senses a rise in blood glucose and tells the pancreas to once again release insulin.

"TROUBLE TRIGGERS": A GUIDE TO DECIPHERING WHEN AND WHY METABOLISM B PROGRESSED

Until your Metabolism B progressed to the point that symptoms kicked in, your body appeared to respond to food like everyone else's, and most reasonable diets worked for you. At some point, however, your metabolism seemed to change. You were born with this genetic predisposition or potential for excess insulin release, insulin resistance, and resultant glucose issues, but for a good chunk of your life, you coasted along without a clue. Although we don't know exactly why the symptoms progress, research indicates that certain events may help set off the progression of Metabolism B.

Triggers that may be responsible for the onset of Metabolism B's symptoms include:

1. *Hormonal change.* Growth spurts, puberty, pregnancy, and menopause all cause dramatic hormonal shifts in your body.

2. *Stress.* Stressful challenges involved with adolescence, the college years, entering the adult workforce, marriage, children, career, divorce, death of a loved one, or aging may trigger Metabolism B.

3. *Illness and pain.* A bad flu virus, surgery, back injury, broken bones, childbirth, severe arthritis, fibromyalgia, cancer, or chronic illness often appears to be the catalyst for Metabolism B's progression.

4. *Medications.* Certain medications for high blood pressure, such as beta-blockers, as well as steroids such as cortisone and prednisone, can cause increases in blood glucose.

5. *Overweight.* The strain of excess body fat and increasing insulin resistance can tax the body's responses.

6. *Physical inactivity.* Exercise helps to decrease blood sugar and insulin release.

THE TIMELINE OF METABOLISM B

Now that you know of Metabolism B, it's helpful to look back over your life and assess when the symptoms for alternate metabolism came to the surface.

Put a check next to the time when your metabolism appeared to shift gears, and you'll find that from that point on, your weight issues, symptoms, and medical history began to change.

☐ As a child, you were either painfully thin or had a pudgy roll around the tummy. There was no "average" weight in your childhood.

☐ Despite your being pencil thin or slightly chubby as a child, your weight changed during your teens or midtwenties. You could no longer get away with dietary indiscretions and could gain five pounds in one weekend! You noticed that although you ate less than your friends, you were always heavier than they were.

☐ If you're a mother, you experienced extreme frustration when trying to lose weight after childbirth. After each delivery, weight loss became even more difficult.

☐ If you're a woman, you noticed a change in weight (even if you were never pregnant). You feel stressed, overwhelmed, and rushed, with less time for exercise and relaxation.

☐ If you're a man, you noticed that you began to develop a midline paunch. Later, you had difficulty buttoning your bottom shirt button, and your waist size increased from 32 to 34 to 36 and up. Work and family obligations took precedence over time spent working out.

☐ Eventually, weight-loss methods that successfully knocked off five or ten pounds in the past stopped working. The older you got, the harder it became to lose weight. At some point, you seemed to lose the battle and cross the line and give up.

☐ No matter what diet program you tried, your excess weight never came off and stayed off. Your friends made diet changes and got results; you made the same changes and gained weight!

☐ Your overall health began to change, and you needed medication for weight-related health problems. You decided to buy a pill box!

☐ You began to feel much older than your age. Your face looked puffy, and there were bags under your eyes. You felt bloated, especially after eating

(continued on page 32)

The Common Eating Habits of Metabolism B

Over the years, I've met thousands of people with Metabolism B. When they sit down in my office to tell their story, it always amazes me how many eating habits they share. See if you recognize yourself in any of these common descriptions.

- Very often, the first point that my patients want to convey is that they don't eat the amount of food that should equal the weight on the scale. Doctors and nutritionists have accused them of underreporting food consumption, closet eating, purging, or outright lying on their diet recall!

- People with Metabolism B have a history of yo-yo dieting and can recall losing and regaining hundreds of pounds throughout their lifetime. They feel frustrated, ashamed, and despondent.

- The breakfast bomb: Half of these patients aren't hungry in the morning and cannot possibly eat breakfast. The other half cannot function without eating in the morning. It's all or nothing regarding the first meal of the day!

- Those who do eat breakfast crave carbohydrates. They seek combinations of toast, bagels, orange juice, cereal with milk, Danish, muffins, doughnuts, and fruited yogurt.

- They feel that they are in "their best control" before they eat anything for the day. They report feeling hungrier once they begin to eat.

- Metabolism B patients often report needing to eat two or three hours after a meal. Midmorning, late afternoon, and nighttime cravings and snacking are very common. When they hold off on eating, they may get cranky, nauseated, or light-headed.

- After lunch, people with Metabolism B frequently feel drowsy and need a nap. They also report craving chocolate, a salty/crunchy snack, or caffeine in the afternoon.

- Most patients with Metabolism B relate needing a caffeine "lift" in the morning or late afternoon. They drink coffee, tea, iced tea, caffeinated soft drinks, energy drinks, or chocolate to pick up their energy.

- Although they'd like to prepare a balanced dinner, these individuals list demanding careers, dual-career families, family commitments, and fatigue among the reasons that they dine out or bring in dinner. Many report having pizza, Chinese food, deli food, fast food, or take-out dinners at least twice a week.

- When eating out, most of these patients try to ignore the bread basket, but once they begin sampling it, they have a difficult time controlling their consumption of bread and rolls.

- Most don't eat dessert as part of dinner but seem to have a "craving" for sweets in the course of the evening. Ice cream is a favorite nighttime snack.

- Pasta can cause a major problem for the Metabolism B patient. Most admit to eating several full plates for the meal, snitching some as they clear the table, picking at the pasta in the refrigerator throughout the evening, and even digging into the pasta bowl in the morning.

- Many people with Metabolism B feel fixated on food, daydreaming about it throughout their day and even thinking about what they are going to eat for dinner as they eat their breakfast.

- Many report sleepiness after eating their nighttime meal and falling asleep in a chair watching the evening news. They wake up a little later in the evening, starving, and begin their nighttime snacking.

- A significant number wake up hungry in the middle of the night. Some get out of bed and head to the refrigerator at 2:00 or 3:00 a.m. for a snack.

- Almost every Metabolism B patient I counsel reports eating more when under stress. These patients typically can't stop snacking when they are stressed.

Interestingly, when your Metabolism B is correctly treated, the eating patterns that were your way of life lessen or even disappear. People cannot believe that the foods they used to crave and look forward to eating no longer have that effect on them. It turns out that the food wasn't that "delicious"; it just provided the necessary blood glucose boost and literally gave comfort. When blood sugar stays in the normal zone, without peaks and valleys, these foods become like any other food.

a meal, and you needed to unbutton your jeans to breathe. You began to feel a variety of aches and pains, and you felt tapped of energy. Mild depression and bouts of anxiety entered your life. You slept fitfully and woke up tired.

☐ Your carbohydrate addiction got worse. You opened the kitchen cabinets and went from bag to carton, bingeing on carb foods. After opening a bag of chips or cookies, you kept returning for more than you intended. You began to worry that you had lost control. Why did you lack the willpower?

REAL READER SUCCESS STORY
Marlene Malloy

Since 2007, Marlene has lost thirty-three pounds.

Favorite MM Recipes: Pasta-Free Veggie Lasagna (page 290), Chocolate Brownie Muffins (page 312)

Marlene's journey started in June 2004, when she began to train for a half marathon for a charity organization. "On the first day of training, they wanted us to run/walk three miles," she says. "As I spent the rest of the day on the sofa not able to move, I asked myself, 'What happened to you?'"

Over the next three years, Marlene trained hard and completed thirteen half marathons and one full marathon while following a conventional meal plan. "I lost twenty pounds, but I couldn't figure out why it was taking so long," she says. "Then someone suggested reading Diane's book, and I thought, 'So that's my problem—I have Metabolism B!'

"It's one of the best and easiest programs I have followed, but you still have to work at it." Before Marlene started the program, she had begun going to the gym at 5:00 in the morning before work five days a week, but it was only after starting Step One that she saw a difference in her weight. Even more than that, she noticed after the first week that she was more focused, slept better, and had more energy.

"Within the first week, I noticed two things: First, I didn't realize how much and how often I ate carbs. Second, after my body reset itself, I didn't want them anymore!" she says. "In the past, whenever the scale would go down, it would be permission to eat. Now I don't have cravings, and for me that is huge! You have no idea what a miracle it has been for me personally to be able to stroll down the baked goods aisle and not be tempted. The Metabolism Miracle gave me the ability to have total control."

Marlene even got her husband in on the act. He started following the diet, too (mostly—he can't give up beer), and lost thirty pounds. "Even though he's Metabolism A, he still benefits from the program," she says. In the beginning, he thought his switch to the Metabolism Miracle would be temporary, but Marlene says that he loves it so much, he hasn't stopped. Together they pore over cookbooks, looking for low-carb recipes. Thanks to the eating plan, they eat far more vegetables than they used to. "I would have never eaten cauliflower before. Asparagus? Ugh—please," she groans. "But you know, now I eat them, and they're really good!

"I'm feeling great, I sleep better, and people compliment the coloring of my skin and say I look like I'm in my twenties. I'm healthy, and when I last had my labs done, the doctor was thrilled with what she saw—my cholesterol and triglycerides have fallen, and my resting heart rate is very low." Marlene has also dropped clothing sizes along the way, going from an 18 to a 12. "I have finally accepted that I have to listen to my body," she says.

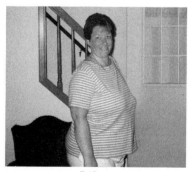

Before

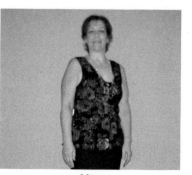

After

Marlene's Advice

"Jump in with both feet. Read the book, read it again, and prepare your kitchen to follow the plan. Clear the cupboard, because if it's not in the kitchen, you won't eat it.

"Your body really does retrain and reset itself. Just know that the scale is the curlicue that Diane talks about. The scale might go up and I just want to cry, but then the following week it will go down. Take a deep breath, go with it, listen to your body, and get on the message board and find friends all over the country."

4

WHAT HAPPENED? "OTHER DIETS USED TO WORK FOR ME"

By now you have a good understanding of how Metabolism B directs your body to store excess blood sugar in your fat cells. The Metabolism Miracle will help to temper your pancreas, calming the insulin release and fat production so that permanent weight loss can occur. But why wouldn't any diet help you to lose weight?

When your friends with Metabolism A want to lose weight, they can follow any reasonable diet because their metabolism follows the classic formula found in any basic nutrition textbook:

Calories eaten – calories burned = weight

In other words, your friends who have metabolism A will gain weight if they consume more calories than they burn off. But they will lose weight if they cut back on total calories while increasing their physical activity. Your friends' cholesterol is determined by their weight, physical activity, and intake of fatty foods. Their triglycerides may increase because of excess alcohol or certain medications, or their blood pressure may increase from excess weight or sensitivity to sodium. However, your weight, cholesterol, triglycerides, blood pressure, and blood sugar are all linked to hormonal imbalance and excess fat storage.

You now know that your metabolism is very different. The law of calories doesn't apply to people with Metabolism B. You may eat far fewer calories than your friends and lose weight initially, but because your body stores excess blood sugar as fat, a diet based on calories will never work for you long term. Your weight, midline fat, and cholesterol are not entirely the result of excess calories or inadequate physical activity. They are caused by the hypermetabolism of carbohydrate and blood glucose being stored excessively in fat cells.

"HELP ME, DOC!"

Most people with Metabolism B have been told by their physician, "You need to lose twenty pounds"—or even more. Naturally, you are very aware that you need to lose twenty pounds, but, despite all of your attempts, you can't seem to make it happen. If you have hypertension, you hear "Cut down on salt and lose some weight." When your cholesterol rises, you hear "Reduce fats and lose some weight." If you progress to diabetes, the advice changes only slightly: "Watch your sugar intake and lose some weight." Unfortunately, that's the extent of the nutrition advice that many patients hear. They leave the doctor's office with a handful of prescriptions, a diet sheet, and a follow-up appointment date. The doctor doesn't have the key to successful weight loss for people with Metabolism B.

In an effort to get some answers, some patients seek out a registered dietitian (RD) and leave that appointment with a copy of the same 1,500-calorie low-fat/low-cholesterol/low-salt playbook that the RD uses for everyone in your condition. But all these patients' hard work to follow the directions from both a doctor and a nutritionist yields little weight loss. Why? Because, if they have Metabolism B, this standard diet, based on "calories in" minus "calories out," will never work for them!

MISGUIDED GUIDELINES

The medical community has known for at least twenty years that many of us have this combination of symptoms that make up what I refer to as Metabolism B. They include difficulty losing weight, overrelease of insulin, blood sugar problems, insulin resistance, metabolic syndrome, high cholesterol and blood pressure, fatigue, depression, carb cravings, and more. And although books have been written to address specific symptoms—diets for insulin resistance or metabolic syndrome, for example—no one has combined the symptoms to successfully tackle them as a group. This is how *The Metabolism Miracle* differs from every other weight-loss book currently available.

None of the medical associations responsible for setting diet guidelines have yet adapted an effective diet and lifestyle plan for the population with Metabolism B. Meanwhile, the old diet guidelines may end up harming rather than improving the weight and health of people with this alternative metabolism.

Please understand that the foundations for traditional diet guidelines were laid before Metabolism B had been identified. They were, in fact, the very guidelines that I depended upon to counsel my patients before I researched the basis for my Metabolism Miracle program. Now that we understand Metabolism B, it astounds me how misguided some of the medical establishment's guidelines continue to be.

Everyone recognizes the USDA food pyramid, with its base of starches and grains. But think about it—that bottom-heavy section encourages us to choose more than half of our daily food from *carbohydrate!* For years, the American Diabetes Association has recommended that from 50 to 55 percent of calories consumed daily by people with diabetes (all of whom have Metabolism B) should come in the form of carbohydrate! The American Medical Association and the American Heart Association recommend low-fat/low-cholesterol diets (by nature higher in carbohydrate) for anyone with heart disease.

This type of carbohydrate-dense diet logic made sense when we thought that only Metabolism A existed. But we now know that a large portion of the population, including the majority of people with diabetes and heart disease, has Metabolism B, and, unless they work with their bodies to handle carbohydrate normally, they store much of their blood sugar as fat rather than use it as energy. No wonder patients with heart disease who follow low-fat/low-cholesterol diets can rarely get their lipids to decrease and must instead depend on statins and other medications to control hypertension and cholesterol.

Recommending that people with Metabolism B, who have trouble processing carbohydrate, consume at least half of their calories from carbohydrate is like advising people with an allergy to dairy to consume half of their daily calories from dairy foods!

For someone with Metabolism B, a higher-carb diet causes cholesterol, triglycerides, blood pressure, and weight to increase! If people with Metabolism B follow these misguided guidelines without first correcting an overreaction to carb, their pancreases will churn out excess insulin and may even begin to tire. These people will gain weight and may require increased doses of medication, and many will become prediabetic or even develop type 2 diabetes. Look around you—the country really is becoming heavier and sicker.

THE "CARB IS A CARB" MYTH

Perhaps you've heard the mantra "A carb is a carb." It is the basis for yet another dietary myth. This is the theory behind carbohydrate counting, which maintains that every carbohydrate gram you eat will eventually turn

Why Other Diets Have Failed You

You probably have a long history of trying diets that work for a while but ultimately fail to keep weight at bay, no matter how closely you follow the rules. The bottom line is that Metabolism B won't respond to the traditional formula for weight loss, which depends upon eating fewer calories than you burn off in a day. This list explains why these popular diets fail anyone with Metabolism B.

Traditional weight-loss program: This approach, based on decreasing the calories you consume while increasing the calories you burn, cannot work for those with Metabolism B because their weight is determined in great part by their response to carbohydrate and blood sugar rise, not simply calories in/calories out.

Low-fat and low-cholesterol diets: When you restrict fat grams, you automatically restrict many protein foods such as red meat, cheese, and peanut butter. With restrictions of both protein and fat, carbohydrate is left to fill the gap. For people with Metabolism B, excess carbohydrate stimulates excess insulin that then stores the carbohydrate glucose as fat. Imagine struggling to follow a low-fat and low-cholesterol diet and watching your cholesterol rise!

Low-carb diet program: Although low-carb diets can often produce an initial weight loss, when carbohydrate is reintroduced without regard to amount, type, or timing, a

into blood sugar and so . . . "a carb is a carb." This misconception has wreaked havoc for people with Metabolism B and is one of the reasons that traditional carb-counting diets will not work for people with alternative metabolism.

To illustrate the theory, consider that both one slice of whole wheat toast and two regular-size chocolate chip cookies contain 15 grams of carbohydrate. Carbohydrate counting asserts that you may choose the carbohydrates you need from *any* category: fruit, milk, starch, or sweets. According to the theory, your blood sugar will rise equally after you consume either the whole grain toast or the cookies. The problem with this philosophy is that different carbohydrates change into blood sugar at different speeds and with different intensities.

When you eat the two cookies, your blood sugar will immediately increase with a sharp spike. By contrast, the whole wheat toast, or any carbohydrate that is naturally high in fiber and low in added sugar, will change to blood sugar at a slower speed without the intense spike.

Metabolism B dieter immediately overreacts to the blood sugar rise, and weight gain is almost instantaneous. Also, a typical low-carb diet does not completely rest the liver from self-feeding every five hours. (See "The Beast Within," page 24.) As a result, when you limit carb or skip a meal, the liver will step up to the plate and release glycogen stores for energy. For those with Metabolism B, the pancreas will overrespond with insulin to enable excess glucose to enter fat cells and generate weight gain!

Very low-calorie diet (VLCD): These medically supervised liquid diets, containing only 500 to 800 calories per day, put the body into a starvation mode. After an initial weight loss, your brain perceives that it is getting too few calories to maintain normal life functions and keep you alive, so it slows metabolic rate to preserve every morsel you consume. At the same time, the Metabolism B pancreas continues to overrespond to blood sugar from carbohydrates and from the liver's release of glycogen. As soon as the dieter reverts to even a low 1,000 calories (most people need more than 1,400 calories), his or her weight begins to balloon.

Fad diets: Diets that focus on magic potions such as cabbage soup, grapefruit, crackers and water, chocolate, or foods of one color will not work for anyone long term. But you already knew that, right?

Low-impact carbohydrates such as brown rice or whole-grain bread have more staying power; they do not prompt the pancreas to release a quick flood of insulin. Instead, their slower release of blood sugar prompts a slower release of insulin. In the medical world, a carbohydrate's impact is determined by its *glycemic index*, which rates how rapidly a carb turns into glucose. In *The Metabolism Miracle*, we'll simply tag carbohydrates with the terms *low impact* and *high impact*.

You can see how the "a carb is a carb" myth becomes a problem. When someone with Metabolism B chooses high-impact carbs such as cookies, they

The Wake-Up Call

Sometimes people who have followed all of their doctors' advice and look like the picture of health have a frightening wake-up call. That's when understanding that they have Metabolism B becomes a matter of life or death.

George loves life. He has been married for over thirty years and has a grandson with whom he enjoys fishing. The fifty-seven-year-old works hard and looks forward to retirement, when he plans to read, walk, fish, and fish—the man loves to fish!

He saw his cardiologist yearly for high cholesterol, walked daily, took his prescribed medications, and followed his low-fat/low-cholesterol diet. When he grilled, he used superlean sirloin, skinless chicken, and fish. He snacked on fat-free pretzels and whole-grain crackers. His potato salad was fat free, and he used frozen fruit bars for dessert. He was determined, despite his high cholesterol, to watch his first grandchild grow up.

But two years ago a heart attack shook up his world.

No one expected cardiac problems in a man who was so careful, so cautious, and so health-conscious. He entered my office scared, explaining that he didn't know what else he could possibly do to prevent another heart attack.

I listened to George's story and took a good look at this man who had followed the traditional diet guidelines to a T. He had a roll of fat around his middle, despite daily exercise and his diet. He took medications for blood pressure, cholesterol, acid reflux, and anxiety. He complained of fatigue and feeling sleepy after meals. He told me that over the past few years, he hadn't felt like himself—that something felt "off."

tax their insulin response much more than if they were to eat exactly the same number of carbohydrates but in a low-impact form, such as the whole wheat bread.

When you have Metabolism B, you must toss out the old carbohydrate myths to achieve permanent weight loss and avoid health issues down the road. It took me a long time to figure out how to save myself from the black hole of textbook diets, but, like my patients who have followed the Metabolism Miracle program, I have kept off weight, improved my health and well-being, and now have boundless energy.

He couldn't sleep well; he woke up tired; and, although he loved his wife, his libido had declined. In fact, his level of joy had also decreased. He couldn't keep up with his grandson, and he even admitted to being less interested in fishing!

His father had died of a heart attack at the age of sixty, and George's own lab report was telling: His glucose was 112 (normal is 65–99 mg/dL [3.6–5.5 mmol/L]), and his LDL cholesterol, triglycerides, and blood pressure were all higher than normal. In fact, he was prediabetic without knowing it.

I explained that the low-fat/low-cholesterol diet was high in the carbohydrate that probably caused his alternative metabolism to overprocess blood glucose into fat. The diet he had so faithfully followed was working against him and may even have been a contributing factor to his heart attack.

George was so entrenched in the low-fat/low-cholesterol diet that he found it difficult to shift gears. His lean protein choices and heart-healthy fat intake were a perfect backdrop for the Miracle program, but he had to make adjustments to his intake of carbohydrates. He was a desperate man, and he wanted his future and life back.

Eight weeks after he began the Metabolism Miracle, George returned, having lost four inches of fat off his belly. His blood pressure, LDL cholesterol, and triglycerides had all improved. He felt energetic and confident and was thrilled with the ease of the program. He left the office with a spring in his step and told me that his fishing pole was already in his car!

REAL READER SUCCESS STORY
Lynn Merit

Since October 2009, Lynn has lost thirty-seven pounds.

Favorite MM Recipe: Lemony Scallop and Shrimp Soup (p. 262)

Before starting the Metabolism Miracle program, Lynn was on the road to diabetes. Her cholesterol and blood sugar numbers ran high, she wasn't sleeping well, and she contended with a frightening family history—both her mother and sister had died at age forty-six, possibly due to similar metabolic problems.

In fall 2009, she read about the Metabolism Miracle and decided she needed to try it. "Committing to MM has been one of the most profound experiences of my life. MM has transformed my well-being not only on a physical level but on an emotional level as well," she says. "It was a godsend to me."

She first noticed changes within three weeks. Her clothes were getting looser, and friends and family took notice, too. "I had someone say, 'Gosh, you've lost so much weight—are you sick?' I told them no— that I've never felt better in my life."

Getting started wasn't hard, Lynn says, but it did force her to take a critical look at her lifestyle: "After forty-nine years of not knowing any better, it was a whole new way of thinking, a whole new way of eating." For example, she learned that she hadn't been drinking enough water and that she needed to include supplements in her diet. "I could go all day without drinking, so really forcing myself to drink water was something I had to add into my life," she says. To keep herself organized, she created her own food log to track her meals, vitamins, and water intake.

Exercising was another area that needed improvement. She began doing cardio and strength-training at the gym, but some of her favorite activities have nothing to do with treadmills and dumbbells. At home, she'll switch on her iPod and dance while doing chores. She also gets moving while walking the beaches near her home in Connecticut with her metal detector. "I metal-detect year-round, and I do it in the water, so I get resistance from the waves. There's a lot of walking, swimming, scooping, and digging," she says. When it's too frosty outside for a beach hunt, she gets a workout by shoveling snow.

Thanks to a new active lifestyle and her success on Steps One and Two of the eating plan, Lynn celebrated her fiftieth birthday this year with friends and family. Her party theme was Hawaiian luau— featuring all MM foods, of course!

Lynn's Advice

First, get focused: "If you're just starting out, don't even read Step Two. Just make sure you understand Step One."

Second, get organized: "Figure out what you need in order to follow Step One and make it available. You might falter if it's not in arm's reach."

Third, think ahead: "Get a support group. Join Diane Kress's support group on Facebook so you can be part of a community that will be supportive and helpful. Don't let family members and friends sabotage your efforts. It's really an easy plan that can change your life. It's going to make you feel so much better."

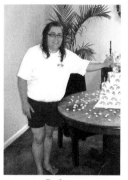
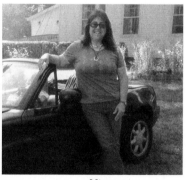

Before   After

PART TWO

A 3-Step Plan to Weight Loss That Will Stay Off

5

STEP ONE—CARB REHAB: EIGHT WEEKS TO A NEW LIFE

STEP-ONE BASICS

TIME: Eight weeks

THE CHALLENGE: A low-carb period to rest your over-worked pancreas and liver while shrinking fat cells

RESULTS: Your energy will soar and you'll feel content. You will lose weight and your belly fat will slim down. Meanwhile, cholesterol, triglycerides, blood sugar, and blood pressure all decrease.

Think of Step One of the Metabolism Miracle as spring cleaning. You will eat many of your favorite foods on this easy, straightforward step, but you will also, in essence, clean up the metabolic mess that has taken control of your body.

For the eight weeks of Step One, you will cut out most carbohydrates from your diet. This will give your pancreas a long-overdue vacation so that it can regroup and reprogram to handle carbohydrates healthily. As you rest your overworked system, your body will create a clean slate for a future at the weight at which you look and feel your best.

As a registered dietitian, I was never a fan of low-carb diets. I felt that there was something wrong with eliminating an entire group of nutrients from the daily diet. Carbohydrate is the preferred fuel for the body. So how could eliminating it be healthy?

After years of researching Metabolism B, I changed my mind. As it turns out, there is only one way to nonmedically control the blood glucose imbalance that plagues people with this alternative metabolism. The program must *temporarily* eliminate most carbohydrates from the diet. This rehabilitative state accomplishes two things:

1. *By eliminating carb-dense foods, you stop contributing sugar to your bloodstream.*

2. *The temporary elimination of most carbs will enable the liver to deplete most of the glycogen stores it uses for the self-feeding mechanism.*

As a result, for the first eight weeks of Step One, your blood sugar will run smoothly, with no spikes that would stimulate the pancreas to overrelease insulin. Your pancreas and liver will take a much-needed temporary vacation to rest and rejuvenate.

A very low-carb diet is not nutritionally balanced, but, as a *temporary* choice to reset a healthy metabolism, it works well by deliberately leaving the pancreas and liver in a state of rest. Carbs come back into the picture on Steps Two and Three, but by then you have established a new metabolic balance that your body can work with beautifully.

THE THREE-DAY KICKER

By the fourth day of Step One, you will be delighted with the changes that your body feels. But the first three days of Step One will be tough—the very reason I've nicknamed this step "rehab" or "detox." Realize that your body has been using carbohydrate for fuel since the day you were born. Now you are asking your brain to choose an alternative fuel source for a short time. Give yourself a few days to acclimate to this new approach. Rome wasn't built in a day.

For the first three days, you can expect to feel tired, cranky, hungry (even as you eat plenty of food), carb-crazed, slightly shaky, light-headed, and a little headachy. Hold on—*you can do it.*

After three days, you will begin to feel much better, with more energy, no hunger, and no carb cravings. You will also be less irritable and much more relaxed. Within a week, once this step is in full swing, you will have no carb cravings, and your friends and family will probably mention how pleasant you are to be around.

Why are those first three days so difficult? Recall that your liver contains a three-day stockpile of blood sugar in the form of glycogen. When you begin Step One and cut out dense carbohydrate from your diet, your liver will feed you with a meal's worth of glycogen around the clock every five hours. That's almost five meals per day! In response to each of those meals, your pancreas will overrelease insulin and your blood sugar will continue to ride a roller coaster, even though you will not be eating much carb. Those blood sugar highs and lows will initially make you irritable and cranky.

At the end of Step One's first three days, as you continue to eliminate blatant carbohydrates and your liver remains purposely depleted of most of its glycogen stores, your brain will have to come up with an alternative plan for fueling the body. As long as you continue to eliminate carbs and your liver remains depleted of glycogen, the brain will choose between consuming muscle or fat for the body's energy needs.

Exercise plays an important role in the Metabolism Miracle, as it literally energizes and activates muscle. The brain will leave active muscle cells alone and focus on consuming the inactive fat cells for energy needs.

Step One is setting up the body exactly as we want it for the next eight weeks, to:

- Retain muscle
- Derive energy from fat
- Consume fat circulating as excess cholesterol and triglycerides
- Rest the overworked pancreas and liver

Your metabolism will begin to adjust to a more stable blood sugar, and, miraculously, your body will consume fat like never before.

To maximize your success and keep yourself in tip-top health, it is important that you follow ten easy guidelines while on the program. Once you

Find Your Baseline

Before you begin Step One, take stock of what you're starting with by noting your weight and body measurements (chest, waist, hips, and more—see pages 161 to 162 in chapter 10 for specific directions). Try to resist remeasuring or reweighing until the very last day of Step One's eight weeks. You will be spared the frustration of the roller-coaster weight loss that characterizes Metabolism B, and you will be ecstatic when you see the final results.

weave them into your life and feel the difference that they make, you'll understand why I call them "Rules to Thrive By." See chapter 8 for more on these guidelines.

1. *Drink at least 64 ounces of water and caffeine-free fluids daily.*

2. *Avoid gaps of more than five hours without a meal or snack.* Spread your food intake throughout the entire day and even into the night. Within one hour of waking up and right before bed, be sure to have a meal or snack.

3. *Take the recommended vitamins, minerals, and supplements.*

4. *Choose nonnutritive sweeteners with care.* I recommend the use of sucralose or stevia as a sugar substitute.

5. *Judge the carbohydrate content of packaged foods by reading the Nutrition Facts section of food labels and using "the formula."* (See "Easy Carb Counting," page 55.)

6. *Consider drinking green tea daily.*

7. *Increase your physical activity to include a minimum of thirty minutes, five times per week.*

8. *Eat allowed foods liberally, but not to excess.*

9. *Practice relaxing.* Take a few minutes each day to close your eyes, breathe deeply, shed your stress, and clear your mind.

10. *Think positively!* First thing in the morning and the last thing at night, remind yourself of your good health, weight loss, high energy level, continuing progress, and positive future.

SIMPLE, SIMPLE, SIMPLE

Perhaps the best part about Step One, besides the fat loss and energy boost, is its ease and simplicity. During Step One, foods fall into two categories: yes and no. People find these food choices incredibly easy to make.

Look at the arrow sheet in this chapter. Each of the four arrows represents a category of foods: lean proteins, healthy fats, allowed vegetables, or carbohydrates. During the eight weeks of Step One, you may eat liberally from the first three arrows, but you must avoid the foods in the carbohydrate arrow. The foods in the protein, fat, and allowed veggie arrows don't require a carb check. You won't need to read food labels for the carb content of nuts, cheese, cottage cheese, or broccoli. Only the carb-containing foods that are starred or marked "5 × 5" carbs require a label check. These foods must be limited to 5 grams in a five-hour period and include low-carb bread, low-carb yogurt, low-carb milk, and the like.

Although most foods contain a combination of nutrients, they are classified into their arrow by the main nutrient that they contain. For example, flank steak and chicken fall into the protein arrow, olive oil and nuts fall into the fat arrow, and white potatoes fall into the carbohydrate arrow.

Sometimes, however, foods can be deceptive. Take the two dairy foods cheese and yogurt. Cheese contains mostly protein, so it fits into the protein arrow. Low-fat yogurt contains protein and fat, but its main nutrient is carbohydrate, so this dairy product is in the carbohydrate arrow.

Many people are surprised to learn that milk, fruit, carrots, and lentils also fit into the carbohydrate arrow. Foods in the carb arrow will have a dramatic impact on blood sugar and cause your pancreas to quickly release insulin. You must avoid these foods during Step One. Not even a pinch.

There is no need to weigh, measure, count, or plot foods from the lean protein, healthy fat, and vegetable arrows. These foods will not stimulate the insulin roller coaster. You can eat them whenever you wish.

You'll notice a small horizontal arrow labeled "5 × 5 carbs." Although typical breads, crackers, yogurts, and other carbohydrate-dense foods must be avoided during Step One, the food industry has come up with low-carb versions of these foods that fit sparingly into Step One. I'll explain this on page 000.

Consider hanging a copy of the "Arrow Sheet" on your refrigerator or keeping one at the office or in your bag to remind you of the foods to avoid on Step One and those that you may eat freely.

CARB CONTROL

The key to Step One is carbohydrate control. You won't eliminate all carbohydrate foods from your diet, but you'll temporarily avoid most of them. The

(continued on page 54)

THE ARROW SHEET

Fat Foods to Enjoy During Step One (And All Other Steps of the Metabolism Miracle)	Veggies to Enjoy Liberally During Step One (And All Other Steps of the Metabolism Miracle)	Protein Foods to Enjoy During Step One (And All Other Steps of the Metabolism Miracle)
Light or whipped butter	Artichokes and artichoke hearts	Lean meat
Light or tub margarine	Asparagus	Skinless poultry
Light sour cream	Green or wax beans	Fish and shellfish
Light mayonnaise	Bean sprouts	Low-fat cheese
Light creamer	Broccoli	Low-fat cottage cheese
Light half-and-half	Brussels sprouts	Eggs
Oils	Cabbage	Egg substitutes
*Light salad dressing	Cauliflower	Natural peanut butter
Olives	Celery	Nut and seed butters
Avocados	Cucumbers	Tofu
Nuts	Dill pickles	*Unsweetened soy milk
Seeds	Eggplant	*Other soy products
	Onions and scallions	Vegetarian meat substitutes
	Greens (collards, kale, mustard, turnip, spinach)	*Low-carb protein shakes
	Kohlrabi	
	Leeks	
	Mushrooms	
	Okra	
	Peppers (all varieties)	
	Lettuce and other salad greens	
	Radishes	
	Spaghetti squash	
	Sauerkraut	
	Tomatoes (maximum 1/meal)	
	*Tomato salsa	
	*Tomato juice	
	*Vegetable juice	
	Turnips	
	Zucchini and summer squash	

Although meats and cheeses are primarily protein, they vary tremendously in their fat content. The recommended protein sources in the Metabolism Miracle program will be heart healthy and lean. You can feel free to enjoy them all liberally.

Carbs to Avoid in Step One

Bread
Bread products
Pasta
Rice
Crackers, pretzels, chips
Cereal and granola bars
Cereal (hot or cold)
Other grains

Fruit
Fruit juice
Potatoes and sweet potatoes
Carrots
Parsnips
Beets
Legumes (beans and peas)
Winter squash

Pumpkin
Milk
Yogurt
Sweetened beverages
Sweets and desserts
Foods that fail the 5 × 5 net carb test

5 × 5 Carbs (in Step One only, have no more than 5 grams of net carb in a five-hour period) for Step One and All Other Steps of the Metabolism Miracle

*Low-carb bread
*Low-carb tortillas
*Low-carb wraps
*Low-carb crackers
*Low-carb ketchup

*Select sugar-free puddings
*Select sugar-free yogurts
*Select sugar-free smoothies
*Select low-sugar juices
*Low-carb milk

*Carb-controlled protein drinks
*Foods or recipes that contain 5 grams or less of net carb per serving

*All of these items must be put through the net carb formula and must fit into the 5 × 5 rule (see "Easy Carb Counting," page 55).

foods in the protein, fat, and veggie arrows that are not starred do not require a food label check, even though they contain a limited amount of carb.

During any five-hour period of Step One, you may eat 5 grams of carbohydrate. This "5 × 5 rule" allows you to eat limited carb grams without stimulating your pancreas to release insulin.

Any carbohydrate above the 5-gram ceiling—$\frac{1}{2}$ cup sugar-free ice cream with its 10 grams of carb, for example—will alert the pancreas to release insulin and will put you right back into the metabolic chaos your body desperately needs to escape. Keep carb intake under the 5-gram bar and your pancreas will remain in its curative resting state.

So how do you know which foods have 5 grams or less of carbohydrates? The list of carbohydrates that you must absolutely avoid during Step One all exceed the 5-gram limit (see "Carbs to Avoid in Step One," page 53). But a number of carbohydrate foods can be eaten during Step One. I call these foods "5 × 5 carbs" because you can tally their carbohydrate total with a quick, easy formula to decide if they fit the 5 × 5 rule. Any foods that have been starred (*) on the food lists fit into the 5 × 5 category. You must be the judge. Never rely on marketing ploys used on the package to tell you the number of carb grams the product contains. You must do the math.

YOU CAN DO IT

Almost every patient with Metabolism B in my practice who sees the "Carbs to Avoid List" begins to panic. They grow pale, shake their heads, and declare, "There is no way that I can do this for eight weeks!"

Your strong reaction to this list of foods is just one more affirmation that you have Metabolism B. However, you should know that every one of the patients who completed the first three days of Step One completed the remainder of the eight weeks.

Your body desires to run on carbohydrate, but it is built to survive with a mechanism to get you through periods without carb. If there is no carbohydrate, the body will run off the liver's stores of glycogen for three days. On the fourth day, it will begin to burn muscle or fat. Because you will be physically active, the exercise will steer your body to burn fat rather than muscle.

On day four, you will not only shift to fat burning, but your brain will take the edge off the absence of carbohydrates. Imagine you are stranded in the desert without carbohydrates. As long as you continue to avoid carb and stay in the fat-burning mode, your brain will shut down your carb cravings, infuse you with energy, and allow you to think clearly so that you can continue looking for food to survive.

The eight weeks will be a breeze if you follow the 5 × 5 rule and avoid foods containing more than 5 grams of carbohydrate in a five-hour period. In Step One, you have an option to include a 5-gram net carb at each of your meals, at bedtime, and even in the middle of the night. You can do this without interrupting the new peace that your body has found.

EASY CARB COUNTING

It may sound like work to figure out how many carbohydrates any particular food has, but in fact it's quite simple. An easy formula, the net carb formula, is the only one you will need to use during the three steps of the Metabolism Miracle.

The Net Carb Formula

Total carbohydrate grams – dietary fiber grams = net carb grams

To use it, look at the nutrition facts label on any food. The only numbers you need pay attention to are serving size, total carbohydrate grams, and dietary fiber grams. The words "total carbohydrate" will always be in dark, bold type on the label. Beneath them, in lighter type and slightly indented, you will find "dietary fiber," along with a slew of other terms such as "sugar" and "sugar alcohol."

All of these subcategories are included in the total carb grams. Dietary fiber, however, although included in the total carb grams, will never change into blood sugar and tax the pancreas. Instead, it goes through your digestive system unabsorbed. Subtracting the fiber, then, allows you to see all the carb that does affect your blood sugar and insulin release. That is the *net carb* and it is key to keeping your Metabolism B on track.

Nutrition Facts	
Serving Size	
Servings Per Container	
Amount Per Serving	
Calories 0	Calories from Fat 0
	% Daily Value*
Total Fat 0g	0%
Saturated Fat 0g	0%
Trans Fat 0g	
Cholesterol 0mg	0%
Sodium 0mg	0%
Total Carbohydrate 0g	0%
Dietary Fiber 0g	0%
Soluble Fiber 0g	0%
Insoluble Fiber 0g	0%
Sugars 0g	
Protein 0g	
Vitamin A 0% • Vitamin C 0%	
Calcium 0% • Iron 0%	
Phosphorus 0% • Magnesium 0%	

* Percent Daily Values are based on a 2,000 calorie diet. Your daily values may be higher or lower depending on your calorie needs:

		Calories:	2,000	2,500
Total Fat	Less than		0g	0g
Sat Fat	Less than		0g	0g
Cholesterol	Less than		0mg	0mg
Sodium	Less than		0mg	0mg
Potassium			0mg	0mg
Total Carbohydrate			0g	0g
Dietary Fiber			0g	0g

Calories per gram:
Fat 0   •   Carbohydrate 0   •   Protein 0

How to Calculate Net Carbs

Here is an example of how to read a food label and calculate the product's net carbs.

KRAZY KRISPIES CEREAL

SERVING SIZE: ¾ cup

TOTAL CARBOHYDRATE: 22 grams

DIETARY FIBER: 2 grams

Subtract the dietary fiber (2 grams) from the total carbohydrate (22 grams) and you have the net carbs (20 grams) for a ¾-cup serving of cereal:

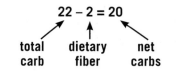

$$22 - 2 = 20$$

total carb   dietary fiber   net carbs

Obviously, with 20 net carbs, this cereal will *not* fit into Step One of the Metabolism Miracle.

Now, let's look at another example:

LOW CARB TORTILLA

SERVING SIZE: 1 tortilla

TOTAL CARBOHYDRATE: 10 grams

DIETARY FIBER: 5 grams

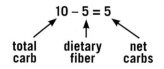

$$10 - 5 = 5$$

total carb   dietary fiber   net carbs

With only 5 net carbs, the tortilla fits into Step One, as long as you remember the 5 × 5 rule and make it the only carb food you eat in a five-hour period of time.

5 × 5 CARBS*

Many people miss breads, crackers, and other traditionally high-carbohydrate foods during Step One of the program. You might consider eating specially designed low-carb versions of these foods, such as the tortilla in our second

* The terms *5 × 5 carbs* and *5 gram "counter" carbs* are used interchangeably in the Metabolism Miracle program.

example. But don't trust the carb count on the front of the package. Instead, always use the net carb formula to determine the carbohydrates in a serving, and remember the 5 × 5 rule. If your low-carb bread comes up at 6 grams of carbohydrate, remove the top crust.

The same goes for a number of starred items in the Step One proteins, fats, and vegetable lists, such as processed peanut butter and prepared salad dressings. You can apply the net carb formula to any foods of which you're unsure, and reduce your serving size accordingly if necessary. The key is simply to stay aware of how many carbohydrates sneak onto your plate.

Unstarred foods in the protein and healthy fat arrow do *not* require a 5 × 5 check. Since cheese, cottage cheese, and nuts are not starred, you need not check their labels for carb content. Consider them to be liberal foods.

Don't make the mistake of stacking carbohydrate foods within the same five-hour period. The 5 × 5 applies to five hours elapsed, total, for foods and beverages consumed. If you choose a 5-gram low-carb wrap for lunch at noon and a 3-gram carb-controlled yogurt for a snack at 2:30 p.m., the combined 8 grams of carbohydrate will exceed the 5 × 5 rule because only two and a

Buyer Beware

Those tempting whole-grain crackers with their "low-carb" label may look like they fit into the 5 × 5 rule, but watch out. Marketing on the front of packages can be deceptively tricky. Food companies have different definitions of "low carb" and "sugar free," and what fits into one low-carb diet may not fit into the Metabolism Miracle diet.

The only way to determine whether the crackers have 5 grams or less carbohydrate and can fit into Step One is to run a serving size through the net carb formula: Total carb—dietary fiber = net carb.

Serving Size: 6 crackers
Total Carbohydrate: 11 grams
Dietary Fiber: 3 grams
11 − 3 = **8 grams**

These crackers do *not* fit into Step One of the Metabolism Miracle. Keep trying—you'll find another product you love that will have 5 grams or less net carb and keep you on the healthy path you've been following.

Sugar Shakedown

Did you know that when you see the word *sugar* on a food label, it refers only to sucrose (table sugar)? All other sweeteners in a food—corn syrup, fructose, or honey, for example—are not included in the "sugar" tally. It is not necessary to look at sugar grams, as sugar is only one small part of the carbohydrate picture. Total carb grams will show you *all* of the carbs in the food item.

half hours have elapsed. The resting pancreas will detect a rise in blood sugar from the 8 grams of carbohydrate and awaken to release insulin, just the outcome you are trying to avoid.

To make life easier, I usually decide if I want a 5 × 5 or starred carbohydrate at breakfast, lunch, dinner, bedtime, and in the middle of the night. I don't use them for between-meal snacks.

WHAT ABOUT SUGAR ALCOHOL?

When reading an ingredient list of products labeled "sugar free," "low sugar," or "low carb," you'll often come across ingredients that end in *ol*, such as mannitol, xylitol, and sorbitol. Ingredients ending in *ol* are most likely sugar alcohols. These ingredients are *not* calorie free. They have less impact on blood glucose than actual sugar because they are not completely absorbed in the GI tract. Because they don't fully absorb, sugar alcohol is known to cause bloating, gas, flatulence, and diarrhea.

Size Matters

Be sure to note the serving size, which can trip you up unexpectedly. Take, for instance, a bottle of flavored iced tea. The 12-ounce bottle looks like one serving, but when you check the nutrition facts label, you see that it is in fact two and half servings. Unless you check the label, you may innocently gulp down the entire bottle with more than twice the carbs you thought you were drinking.

Creative serving sizes can push all of your hard effort on Step One right off track. Keep your eye on the serving sizes when you use the net carb formula.

When you read the Nutrition Facts label, you'll often note "sugar alcohol" under the heading for total carbohydrate. But do not be fooled: Sugar alcohol *does* affect blood sugar and insulin release. It is listed under the total carbohydrate heading because it is partially absorbed as a carbohydrate.

Never subtract sugar alcohol from the total carbohydrate grams when reading a food label. Many companies list a product's net carb grams on its front labeling. The low grams advertised may look temptingly good, but there is a chance that such companies are subtracting both dietary fiber *and* sugar alcohol from the total carbohydrate grams. This is not a legitimate net carb amount because part of the sugar alcohol will affect blood sugar and insulin release. Don't be deceived; read the real ingredient label to get the true picture.

FREE ZONES

Now that you have a sense of the easy carb counting you'll do on Step One, take enjoyment from the fact that you won't have to count a thing in the lean proteins, healthy fat, vegetable, and other "liberal" categories. There is no food weighing, measuring, or counting of "free foods" during Step One. Have them anytime in reasonable quantities and you'll continue to lose weight and feel great.

THE PROTEIN-FAT PACK: MEAT, CHEESE, NUTS, AND MORE

Lean proteins have the green light in the Miracle program, so eat them liberally. Skinless poultry, lean cuts of beef, reduced-fat cheese, egg whites, and

Be Careful with Low-Carb Recipes

The carbohydrate in most "low-carb" recipes exceeds the Step One limit. Even products designed for other low-carb diets will rarely fit into Step One of the Miracle. *When in doubt, stay with the recipes in this book that are permitted for Step One.*

other proteins will provide your body with a sense of satisfaction and staying power. While prime rib and sirloin are both proteins, only the sirloin, because of its low-fat profile, is on the recommended protein list. Your body will always burn the fat from what you have eaten before it will burn your fat stores. The sirloin will help you take full advantage of your body's new fat-burning mode.

A Day in the Life of Step One

Debbie began her first day of the Metabolism Miracle excited about the program that would finally match her body's needs but somewhat anxious about cutting out the carbs. She usually began her day heavy in carbohydrates, with either cereal, a bran muffin, or a bagel. To start her new regimen, she instead had a breakfast of scrambled eggs and low-carb toast with whipped butter. She sipped her coffee and she thought, "I can do this."

As her breakfast digested, the only item that contributed to her blood glucose was the low-carb toast. Debbie's brain barely sensed this tiny rise in blood sugar (and since the toast contained only 5 grams of carb, her brain didn't call on the pancreas for an insulin release). Within two hours of eating her breakfast, Debbie heard the coffee cake on the counter calling her name.

She remembered my telling her to stay strong and ignore the cravings for the first three days. She grabbed a handful of almonds and went on with her day.

Right before lunch, Debbie got very hungry. She longed for the cold pizza slice in the refrigerator, but she heard me say, "Ignore the cravings, eat anything on the free list, and move on." So she grabbed a low-carb wrap, filled it with lean roast beef and Lorraine Swiss, lettuce, tomato, and a dab of mayo, and called it lunch. She was filled up and felt, "I can do this."

As the afternoon wore on, Debbie got very tired. She yearned for some chocolate and a nap. She realized that this was her brain trying to get her to give in and take some preferred fuel—carbohydrate. She reassured herself, ate a spoonful of peanut butter and a protein shake, and went on with her day.

Dinner was no problem. Her energy had returned; she was proud of how well she was doing with her program and was thrilled that Step One required no special

When you choose lean proteins, healthy fats, and vegetables found on the arrow list, you won't have to concern yourself with serving sizes. You can even, on occasion, choose a protein with a higher fat content. Just remember that after day three of your program, your body has transitioned to a fat-burning mode, and you want to take full advantage of that by choosing lean or light proteins so your body won't waste time burning fat from the food. Instead, it will focus on burning your excess fat.

preparation. She sat down with her family to grilled chicken with broccoli, a large salad, and a heaping cup of sugar-free gelatin with light whipped cream for dessert. Life was good.

Things got tough at 9:00 p.m., when Debbie walked into the kitchen. "Mom, can we have popcorn?" "Honey, while you're in there, would you get me some ice cream?"

Debbie muttered under her breath, "Are they crazy? They know I'm watching carbs and they want me to get the carb snacks that they will eat in front of me?" Just when she was about to snap at her family, she remembered, "One step in front of the other for three days, and then hunger and cravings will pass." While the popcorn popped and before she dished out the ice cream, she grabbed a Step One Chocolate Brownie Muffin (recipe on page 312) that she had made earlier in the day. As everyone else snacked, so did Debbie.

Later that night, while her family fell asleep and Debbie had time to read and unwind, she had a cup of Cinnamon Ricotta Pudding (see recipe on page 315) and thought, "I can do this." And she did.

She carried on, maneuvering effortlessly through the next few days and finding it easy, knowing exactly which foods were allowed with no need to weigh or measure them. She indulged in occasional carbs by following the 5 × 5 rule.

Soon, day four arrived. Sure enough, Debbie woke up with a bit more energy, and she couldn't believe that in such a short time, she was accustomed to her program, had eaten a meal in a restaurant with no problem, felt no carb cravings, and had more energy. Debbie continued with Step One for the full eight weeks and looked forward to Step Two.

THE "YES" LISTS

Choose any of these proteins during *any* step of the Metabolism Miracle:

Lean Proteins

POULTRY

Chicken and turkey (white meat, skinless)

Cornish game hen

Be sure to eat poultry without the fatty skin. (Rotisserie chicken, turkey bacon, turkey sausage, and turkey kielbasa all have a higher fat content, so limit their use.)

BEEF

Flank steak	Rib roast
London broil	Porterhouse steak, trimmed
Sirloin	Rump roast
85–93% ground beef	Filet mignon
T-bone steak, trimmed	Chuck roast
Tenderloin	Round steak
Ground round	

Because most people with untreated Metabolism B have elevated cholesterol, they are advised by their physicians or cardiologists to limit red meat. The fact is that lean cuts of red meat are fine to enjoy on a regular basis. USDA Select cuts are leanest, USDA Choice grades have moderate fat, and USDA Prime cuts contain the most fat. In any case, always trim any visible fat.

FISH AND SHELLFISH

Cod	Tuna (fresh or canned in water)
Pollock	Halibut
Trout	Oysters
Swordfish	Whiting
Snapper	Lobster
Mahimahi	Haddock
Flounder	Shrimp
Clams	Sardines
Herring (not creamed)	Scallops
Crab	Sea bass
Tilapia	Imitation shellfish

Eat fish and seafood broiled, grilled, boiled, or steamed, as long as you omit any breading, coating, or cocktail sauce.

PORK

Pork tenderloin	Fresh ham
Canadian bacon	Deli ham
Canned, cured, or boiled ham	Center-cut loin chops
Trimmed pork chops	

Many cuts of pork are lean, but pork "products" such as sausage and patties contain added fat you should avoid.

LAMB, VEAL, AND GAME

Roast lamb	Lean veal chop
Skinless duck	Bison
Lamb chop	Veal roast
Ostrich	Skinless pheasant
Leg of lamb	Venison
Deer	Rabbit

Be sure to trim all visible fat.

CHEESE

Low-fat cheese

Part-skim ricotta, mozzarella, string cheese

Low-fat cottage cheese

Grated cheese, such as Parmesan

Cheese with 5 grams or less fat per ounce

Choose low-fat cheeses and cottage cheese with 1% or 2% milk fat.

I prefer low-fat cheeses over fat-free choices because the latter tends to be plasticlike and refuses to melt. Nutrition fact labeling lists the serving size for cheese as 1 ounce. If cheese has 5 grams or less fat per ounce, it is a low-fat cheese.

You may choose regular cheese, but be aware that your body will spend time burning the fat from the cheese instead of the fat off your body. Be aware when eating out: Restaurants rarely carry low-fat cheeses, so you may choose to have regular cheese when eating out, but stock your home or office refrigerator with the low-fat variety.

EGGS

Whole eggs (maximum 5 yolks/week)

Egg substitute

Eat as many egg whites or as much egg substitute as you like, as they contain no fat. Try to limit your egg yolks to five per week. When making an omelet, for example, use two or three egg whites but only one of the yolks.

SOY PRODUCTS

Tofu

*Vegetarian or soy-based meat

*Unsweetened soy milk substitutes

A half cup (4 ounces) of tofu has as much high-quality protein as an ounce of meat.

When you opt for vegetarian meat substitutes such as veggie burgers or veggie nuggets, use the net carb rule to be sure that they have 5 grams or less per serving. Some veggie products contain hidden carbohydrate from chickpeas, lentils, or kidney beans.

PEANUT AND NUT BUTTERS

Natural peanut butter (refrigerate after opening)

*Processed peanut butter or nut butters (use 5 × 5 rule)

Natural almond butter (refrigerate after opening)

Natural peanut butter, with only peanuts and optional salt as ingredients, offers the best choice during Step One because most processed peanut butter is sweetened with sugar. Just as you don't have to be concerned about the carb content of nuts, you don't have to count the carb in natural peanut butter. Processed peanut butter will require counting as a 5 × 5 food, due to added sugar.

"Sweetened" Peanut Butter

If you miss the taste of your childhood peanut butters, which were often hydrogenated and sweetened, try making your own from natural versions:

1. Remove the top from the natural peanut butter jar.

2. Microwave for about thirty seconds to soften the peanut butter.

3. Stir in two (1 gram) packets of Splenda and, if desired, a pinch of salt.

4. Store in the refrigerator.

*REDUCED-CARBOHYDRATE PROTEIN SHAKES

These premixed ready-to-drink shakes have the protein of about 3 ounces of meat along with added vitamins and minerals. You can find them in the supermarket or pharmacy. Most have only 1 to 3 grams of net carbohydrate.

Heart-Healthy Fats

BUTTER/MARGARINE

Whipped butter

Light butter

Light, tub, and whipped margarines (avoid hydrogenation)

Butter blends (half butter, half oil)

For years, butter has had a bad reputation because it is made from the saturated fat of milk. Margarine is made of vegetable oil, which is not a saturated fat. On the surface, oil seems like a healthier alternative to the use of a saturated fat, right? Wrong. The healthy oil used in margarine was made spreadable by pumping in hydrogen (called *hydrogenation*). This process jarred the oil's fat chains and broke them apart, releasing *free radicals*, trans fats that have been linked to certain kinds of cancer. Note the rise in stomach and colon cancer from the advent of margarine, vegetable shortening, creamy peanut butter, and mass-produced baked goods after the late 1940s.

If you are choosing margarine or spread, you must look for a product that contains no trans fats. Check the ingredient list for *no* partial hydrogenation. The first ingredient should be *liquid* oil, not partially hydrogenated oil.

OILS

Olive oil	Peanut oil
Sunflower oil	Vegetable oil
Canola oil	Safflower oil
Corn oil	

* Starred items must be checked with the net carb formula and must fit into the 5 × 5 rule. (See "Easy Carb Counting," page 55.)

SALAD DRESSINGS

Most regular dressings and true vinaigrettes contain a very small amount of carbohydrate, but vinaigrettes contain even less. Use regular salad dressing in a light amount, to keep your fat intake down without added carbohydrate. The age-old technique of taking salad on your fork and dipping it lightly into your salad dressing on the side really does help to cut down on your total fat consumption.

Avoid fat-free salad dressings. The manufacturer generally replaces the flavor of the fat with sugar, bringing the carb count climb into the danger zone. If you are consuming a lower-fat dressing that contains carb, make sure that the portion you are using is less than 5 grams of carb.

MAYONNAISE

Light or low-fat preferred

OLIVES

Green, black, stuffed

NUTS

Almonds, cashews, pecans, pistachios, and walnuts are all good choices. Also, peanuts, technically legumes, are acceptable. Avoid honey-roasted nuts, however, because honey is a natural sugar coating. If you have a condition called diverticulosis or if you are having stomach or intestinal upset, check with your physician. Some physicians tell these patients to chew nuts into a smooth paste before swallowing, to ease their digestion.

A handful of nuts in the midmorning, midafternoon, and evening can be a great choice of snack. Although they have carbohydrate, the healthy fat content of nuts slows their digestion, and the carbohydrate is released so slowly that it is negligible to your blood glucose. Spread your intake of nuts throughout the day, and don't go overboard with the quantity. I once had a patient who consumed five pounds of pistachios in one afternoon. She called the office in the late afternoon, complaining of stomach pains!

How Much Is Too Much?

Keep in mind that although the majority of your excess weight is due to the over-processing of carbohydrate, large portion sizes of proteins and fats will also contribute to your weight. If you consume excessive quantities of meats and fats, your body will have no choice but to store the excess as fat.

For that reason, unlike some other low-carb diets, the Metabolism Miracle will never suggest that you eat a quarter-pound of bacon, drench your salad in blue cheese dressing, or smother your broccoli with heaping spoonfuls of butter. But you can have Canadian bacon, balsamic vinaigrette, and broccoli with a touch of whipped butter and continue to lose fat and weight.

I once had a patient who took the words "eat liberally" literally. She ate a jar of natural peanut butter a day. I pointed out that although the natural peanut butter was in the protein arrow and not considered a carb in the Miracle program, it *is* a high-fat item. Peanuts and peanut oil, albeit healthy fats, are still fats. So . . . all the while she had followed Step One and steered her body into the fat-burning mode, she had been sabotaging herself by burning the peanut butter's fat! Use common sense and consume normal portions of lean protein, heart-healthy fat, and low-carb veggies.

SEEDS

Sesame, pumpkin, sunflower

Tahini paste (ground sesame seeds; use as a dip or a spread for vegetables)

AVOCADO

Avocado has heart-healthy monounsaturated fats, but keep in mind that one avocado has the fat content of 8 teaspoons of oil!

SOUR CREAM OR CREAM CHEESE

Light or reduced-fat is recommended.

CREAMER OR HALF-AND-HALF

Light or low-fat is recommended. When using flavored creamers, check against the net carb test and count them as a 5 × 5 carb. Regular half-and-half, used lightly because of its high fat content, is also fine.

Neutral Vegetables

Go to town eating the following vegetables. With the exception of tomatoes and tomato products that must be limited (see "Tomato Tip," page 306), you may eat these vegetables at any time and in any quantity, even during Step One. They are filled with vitamins, minerals, fiber, and antioxidants for great health.

Artichoke

Artichoke hearts

Asparagus

Green beans, wax beans

Bean sprouts

Broccoli

Brussels sprouts

Cabbage

Cauliflower

Celery

Cucumber

Dill pickles

Eggplant

Onions and scallions

Greens such as collards, kale, mustard, and turnip greens

Kohlrabi

Leeks

Mushrooms

Okra

Peppers (all colors)

Radishes

Salad greens, including all lettuce, endive, escarole, romaine

Summer squash or zucchini

Spaghetti squash

Sauerkraut

Spinach

Tomato (maximum 1/meal)

Cherry tomatoes (maximum 10/meal)

*Tomato juice (4 ounces/meal)

*Vegetable juice (4 ounces/meal)

*Canned tomatoes (½ cup/meal)

Turnips

*Salsa (½ cup/meal)

You'll notice that certain vegetables, such as carrots, beets, and peas, don't show up on this list. These vegetables contain enough carbohydrate in the amount that will disrupt Step One. Instead, focus on the many veggies above that will keep your pancreas resting and your fat burning.

FREEBIES DURING STEP ONE

During Step One, you can have these foods whenever you like, if their carb grams are zero:

SWEET TREATS

Sugar-free gelatin

Sugar-free chewing gum

Sugar-free ice pops

Sugar-free jelly

Sugar-free syrup

BASICS

Bouillon

Consommé

Broth

BEVERAGES

Club soda

Tea

Diet soda

Select fitness waters, flavored waters, and flavored seltzers

Sugar-free tonic water

Coffee

CONDIMENTS

White horseradish

Vinegar

Lemon and lime juice

Herbs

Mustard

Spices

Dill pickles

The Low-Carb, Low-Sugar Bandit

One brand of ice pop features the Splenda logo. The label states, "Use in low-carb diets," and on the front is declared: "4 grams of net carb!" The pops seem perfect for Step One, right? Look again, this time with the net carb formula to help you:

Serving Size: 1 ice pop
Total Carbohydrate: 12 grams
Dietary Fiber: 4 grams
Sugar: 4 grams
Sugar Alcohol: 4 grams

12 grams (total carb) − 4 grams (dietary fiber) = **8 grams (net carbs)**

Because the pops contain sugar alcohol as well as sugar, the real answer for net carb is not the 4 grams promoted on the front of the package but 8 grams! This product is not allowed on Step One of your diet.

Companies get away with faulty math because the FDA currently has no set formula for net carb. The ice pop manufacturer subtracted both the dietary fiber and the sugar alcohol grams to come up with 4 net carbs listed on the front of the package. But sugar alcohol affects blood glucose, and if you inadvertently slipped this food into your diet on Step One, your pancreas would release insulin and set you back.

Most low-carb products on your store's shelves similarly misrepresent the net carb grams on the front of their packages. *Always* use the net carb formula to protect yourself.

WHAT ABOUT ALCOHOLIC BEVERAGES?

In their unfermented form, grapes and grains pack quite a few carbs. But once fermented or distilled, they chemically change into alcohol that no longer follows the body's carbohydrate pathway. As a result, alcohol does not cause blood glucose to spike in the way carbohydrate would.

During Step One, your liver, the organ that helps to clean alcohol from the bloodstream, is on temporary vacation. While it rests, it may be a bit slower to process alcohol and, as a result, you will feel alcohol's effects faster and for a longer time. So although one or two drinks in a night will probably fit into Step One of the Metabolism Miracle, please drink alcohol wisely and slowly to feel its effect before continuing.

The Buzz on Beer

Regular beer is not allowed on the Miracle program because it contains too much carbohydrate, even after fermentation. Light beer, on the other hand, is processed further and the result is often diluted with water, bringing its carb content into the acceptable range.

Be sure to consult your physician regarding alcohol because certain medications and health conditions such as diabetes can change your reaction to alcohol. On the Metabolism Miracle program, the maximum recommended amount of alcohol (and only with physician approval) is one or two alcohol-containing beverages. A "drink" is defined as:

5 ounces wine

12 ounces light beer

1½ ounces spirits (gin, vodka, whiskey)

STEP ONE SAMPLE MENUS

DAY 1

Breakfast

Egg substitute omelet with chopped peppers, onions, and tomato

1 slice low-carb toast (5 g net carb) with whipped butter and sugar-free jelly

Coffee with half-and-half and Splenda

Midmorning Snack

Handful of almonds

1 piece string cheese

16 ounces flavored water

Lunch

1 low-carb wrap (4 g net carb) filled with sliced turkey breast, sliced cheese, shredded lettuce, tomato, and mayonnaise

Sugar-free gelatin

16 ounces water with lemon

Afternoon Snack

Strawberry protein shake (1 g net carb)

Celery sticks with peanut butter

Dinner

Lean grilled burger

Generous piece of Pasta-Free Veggie Lasagna (recipe on page 290)

Tossed salad with balsamic vinaigrette

Lemon Ricotta Pudding (recipe on page 316)

16 ounces decaffeinated green tea

Nighttime Snacks

Handful of nuts, string cheese, Chocolate Brownie Muffin (recipe on page 312) (5 g net carb)

DAY 2

Breakfast

Vanilla protein shake (1 g net carb)

Handful of almonds

Midmorning Snack

Spoonful of natural peanut butter with celery sticks

Decaffeinated coffee with half-and-half and Splenda

Lunch (ordered from Chinese takeout)

Egg drop soup

Steamed shrimp and vegetables with no sauce (use some of the egg drop soup as "sauce")

Green tea

Afternoon Snack

String cheese and handful of almonds

16 ounces water

Dinner

Grilled chicken Caesar salad (no croutons) with dressing on the side

Low-carb tortilla (5 g net carb)

Sugar-free gelatin with light whipped cream

16 ounces flavored water

Nighttime Snacks

Chocolate Ricotta Pudding (recipe on page 315)

Handful of Parmesan Chips (recipe on page 236)

Breakfast Suggestions for Step One

Egg white omelet with peppers, onions, tomato, and mushrooms, or egg
  white or egg substitute omelet with ham and low-fat Cheddar
1 slice low-carb toast (5 g or less net carb) with whipped butter

4 ounces vegetable juice (5 g or less net carb)
Scoop of low-fat cottage cheese or part-skim ricotta cheese sprinkled
  with walnuts and cinnamon

Low-carb chocolate shake (5 g or less net carb)
Handful of peanuts

Easy Egg Cup (recipe on page 218)
1 slice Canadian bacon
1 slice low-carb toast (5 g or less net carb)

Low-carb yogurt smoothie (5 g or less net carb)
Handful of almonds

1 slice low-carb bread (5 g or less net carb) with melted cheese and
  tomato slices

Low-carb tortilla wrap (5 g or less net carb) spread with natural peanut
  butter

Low-carb yogurt (5 g or less net carb)
Celery sticks with peanut butter

1 slice low-carb bread (5 g or less net carb) spread with low-fat cream
  cheese and sugar-free jelly

Miracle Quiche (recipe page 219)
Zucchini Muffin (5 g or less net carb) (recipe page 314)

6 Silver Dollar Pancakes (recipe on page 225) with whipped butter and
  sugar-free syrup
2 strips turkey bacon

1 slice low-carb toast (5 g or less net carb) with 1 tablespoon natural
  peanut butter
1 cup unsweetened soy milk

1 slice low-carb toast (5 g or less net carb) spread with low-fat ricotta
  cheese and cinnamon; heat in a toaster oven until warm

Take-Out Fake Out

Just because you're restricting carbs doesn't mean you have to cook for every meal. Here are a few take-out solutions that work for any step in the program.

What to choose for Chinese takeout? Appetizer choice: Eat the inside filling of an egg roll (leave the wrapper behind!). Main course: Order steamed broccoli with your choice of shrimp, pork, or beef (no cornstarch or sauce—just steamed!). Then use egg drop soup or chicken broth as a flavorful neutral "sauce" for your entrée.

What to order at a pizzeria? Appetizer choice: Share an antipasto plate or order a side garden salad. Main course: Try a calzone stuffed with any or all of the following: mozzarella, ricotta, ham, onions, bell peppers, and mushrooms. Eat the inside, and leave the outside "crust" behind. You can also order a few slices of pizza with toppings such as grilled chicken, onions, peppers, and cheese; eat the topping of the pizza and leave the crust. If you've got room left for carbs, add a light beer to wash it all down.

Lunch Suggestions for Step One

Tuna salad with light mayonnaise on a bed of crisp lettuce and tomato wedges
Sugar-free gelatin

Italian Vegetable Soup (recipe on page 257)
Chicken Caesar salad without croutons and with Caesar dressing on the side (use sparingly)

Chef's salad with ham, cheese, egg, turkey, and low-fat cheese, with light dressing on the side
Parmesan Chips (recipe on page 236)

Sirloin burger without the bun, with low-carb ketchup and lettuce, tomato, and onion as desired
Side salad with light dressing

Miracle Grilled Cheese (recipe on page 229)
Tomato wedges
Cinnamon Ricotta Pudding (recipe on page 315)

Turkey and light cheese roll-ups with peppers and tomatoes, wrapped in a low-carb tortilla wrap (5 g or less net carb)
Sugar-free gelatin

Low-carb yogurt (5 g or less net carb)
Ham and cheese roll-ups
Celery sticks with peanut butter

Light cottage cheese in a hollowed red bell pepper "cup"
Tossed salad with balsamic vinaigrette
1 slice low-carb toast spread with garlic butter (5 g or less net carb)

Grilled chicken strips over romaine lettuce leaves sprinkled with feta cheese and almonds with light dressing

Italian Vegetable Soup (recipe on page 257)
Turkey/cheese roll-ups
Handful of Parmesan Chips (recipe on page 236)

Shrimp salad with light mayonnaise over a bed of dark greens
Lemon Ricotta Pudding (recipe on page 316)

Chunky Chicken Salad (recipe on page 271) and sun-dried tomatoes on a crisp salad base, with low-fat dressing of choice

1 slice low-carb bread (5 g or less net carb) with natural peanut butter and sugar-free jelly
Celery sticks with cream cheese
Sugar-free gelatin with whipped topping

Easy Pizza (recipe on page 227)
Antipasti: ham, fresh mozzarella, black olives, and tomatoes

Dinner Ideas for Step One

Roasted chicken breast with fat-free gravy (5 g or less net carb)
Mashed Cauliflower (recipe on page 307)
Green beans amandine

London broil with sautéed mushrooms
1 slice low-carb garlic toast (5 g or less net carb)
Tossed salad with light dressing
Broccoli with light cheese sauce

Broiled flounder
Oven-roasted peppers, onions, and zucchini
Mashed Cauliflower (recipe on page 307)
Sugar-free gelatin with whipped topping

Miracle "Spaghetti" (recipe on page 275)
1 slice low-carb garlic bread (5 g or less net carb)
Caesar salad with light dressing

Chicken Paprikash (recipe on page 266)
Steamed green beans
Chocolate Brownie Muffin (recipe on page 312) with light whipped
   cream topping

Chicken broth with "free" veggies
Tender Spinach Salad (recipe on page 247)
Handful of Parmesan Chips (recipe on page 236)
Sugar-free ice pop

Sliced turkey breast with low-fat gravy
Broccoli-Cheese Casserole (recipe on page 298)
"Gilded" Cinnamon Muffin (recipe on page 313)

Pork tenderloin
Roasted vegetables
Tossed salad with light dressing
No-sugar-added pudding (5 g or less net carb)

Sirloin burger on a grilled portobello mushroom (as a bun), with low-fat
   cheese, low-carb ketchup, and lettuce, tomato, and onion
Raw vegetables (no carrots) with low-fat onion dip

Broiled tilapia
Broiled tomatoes with Parmesan cheese
Steamed spinach
Sugar-free gelatin with whipped topping

Turkey hot dogs with mustard in a low-carb wrap (5 g or less net carb)
Sweet-and-Sour Cukes (recipe on page 247)
Sugar-free ice pop

Veggie or meatless burger (5 g or less net carb) and light cheese, open
faced on 1 slice of low-carb bread (5 g or less net carb) with low-carb
ketchup

Cabbage Salad (recipe on page 245)

Grilled Pork Chop
Mashed Cauliflower (recipe on page 307)
Broccoli crowns
Side salad with light dressing
Sugar-free gelatin with whipped topping

Baked chicken breast
Sweet-and-Sour Cukes (recipe on page 247)
Roasted eggplant and peppers
Square of dark chocolate (5 g or less net carb)

Snack Ideas for Step One

Many people choose to use noncarb snacks and save their 5×5 carb choices
for mealtime and bedtime. Remember not to stack carbs during Step One—
you have the option to choose up to 5 grams of net carb in no briefer than a
five-hour period.

Part-skim string cheese
Light-cheese wedges
Low-fat cottage cheese
Nuts
Spoonful of natural peanut butter
Celery sticks with natural peanut butter or light cream cheese
Veggies with light dip
Olives
Turkey or ham and cheese rolls
Low-carb shake (5 g or less net carb)
Protein shake (5 g or less net carb)
Low-carb yogurt or smoothie (5 g or less net carb)
Low-carb or sugar-free hot chocolate (5 g or less net carb)
Sugar-free ice pop
Sugar-free gelatin with whipped topping
Parmesan Chips (recipe on page 236)

Parmesan Chips (recipe on page 236) with salsa (5 g or less net carb)

Meringue cookies (5 g or less net carb)

Ricotta puddings (recipes on pages 315 to 316) (5 g or less net carb)

Crispy Tortilla Chips (recipe on page 235) (5 g or less net carb)

Chocolate Brownie Muffin (recipe on page 312) (5 g or less net carb)

"Gilded" Cinnamon Muffin (recipe on page 313) (5 g or less carb)

Zucchini Muffin (recipe on page 314) (5 g or less net carb)

STEP ONE—FREQUENTLY ASKED QUESTIONS

I got on the scale after seven days on Step One and saw no weight loss. What's going on?

When you begin the Metabolism Miracle, take your starting weight and body measurements (see chapter 10), and don't step back on that scale for at least a full month. Remember, this program not only brings about permanent weight loss but also cleans up excesses in fats and sugar and rests your pancreas and liver. Only after the third day, when your liver has emptied its glycogen stores, will you begin burning excess fat; seven days is too soon to see a change in weight.

Follow the plan, get physically active, take one day at a time, and measure your progress in eight weeks. The results will be worth the wait!

Mozzarella Sticks with Marinara Sauce Dip

Heat ½ cup of marinara sauce in a small single-serving bowl (check the ingredients for no added sugar). Set aside. Remove string cheese from its wrapper, place on a microwave-safe plate, and microwave on high for 5 to 10 seconds to remove its chill. Dip in the warm marinara sauce and smile . . . neutral and *delicioso*.

Don't have a jar of marinara sauce handy? Make your own. A half cup is neutral on all Steps. Choose seasoned diced tomatoes canned in tomato juice (many brands now come mixed with your favorite seasonings, such as garlic, onion, peppers, or basil.) Blend in a food processor with a sprinkle of grated cheese (to thicken). Heat and use as a neutral sauce for string cheese, veggies, shirataki noodles, whole wheat pasta, chicken parm, and more.

For the past eight weeks, everyone has remarked that I look great. I feel rested and energized, and I've tightened my belt three holes. Why does it look like I've lost twice as much as the scale says?

On every other diet plan, you lose a combination of water, fat, and muscle. Steps One and Two of the Metabolism Miracle are fat-burning phases. Fat is light, fluffy, big-volume tissue. When you lose ten pounds of fat, it looks and feels like twenty.

The Miracle leaves what your body needs—muscle and water—and burns excess fat. Your clothes will fit as if you've lost twice the amount, and your lipids, blood pressure, and blood sugar will improve as if you've lost double the scale weight. Celebrate your loss and look forward to more!

Two weeks into Step One, I caved and ate a brownie! What now?

Get back on track right now. The longer you wait, the harder it will be to restart. Continue to count the two weeks you put into the program and begin your next six weeks on Step One. If you really fell out of line, with three or more indiscretions in one week, it would be best to go back to the beginning of your eight-week program.

Just Desserts

The following sweet ideas can quell your sugary cravings on any step of the plan.

Long for a sundae? How about a heaping scoop of Chocolate Ricotta Pudding (recipe on page 315) topped with whipped cream, carb-free chocolate syrup, and chopped walnuts!

Try cottage cheese with a "side" of fruity spread. You've seen the individual ½-cup containers of cottage cheese with a side accompaniment of fruited jam. It's easy to concoct a great substitute for all Steps of the Metabolism Miracle! Cottage cheese is a neutral food (low-fat varieties preferred). Zero-carb fruit-flavored spreads (Walden Farms makes one) have all the sweetness and flavor of regular jam. Just take a spoonful of cottage cheese and dip it in the fruit spread for a delicious after-dinner snack.

I'm constipated during Step One. Help!

You probably aren't drinking the 64 ounces of caffeine-free fluid you need each day. In Steps One and Two, fat-burning phases, your kidneys will cleanse your bloodstream of the breakdown products of fat burning, and your body will flush this waste out with urine. If you don't drink adequate fluid, your body will take needed fluid from your tissues and even your gastrointestinal tract, and you will be left with hardened, difficult-to-pass stools. Even if you aren't thirsty, drink, drink, drink!

Also be sure to keep up your fiber intake with raw vegetables, salads, nuts, and 5 × 5 whole-grain bread products. Two teaspoons of a fiber supplement powder made of powdered plant fiber can add 10 grams of fiber with no extra carb. Finally, exercise is critical to keep things moving along.

I found a pudding marked "Sugar-Free/Use on a Low-Carb Diet." How do I know if it's okay to eat during Step One?

There is only one way to determine if a food is right for Step One. Check the nutrition facts label and do the net carb formula: Total carb grams— dietary fiber grams = net carbs.

If a serving's net carb is less than or equal to 5 grams, it is suitable for Step One.

How many 5-gram net carb foods can I have at a meal?

Use the 5 × 5 rule: Limit yourself to 5 grams of net carb in a five-hour period. I usually suggest that you spread apart your 5 gram net carbs among breakfast, lunch, dinner, and bedtime. When you place them closer, in midmorning or late-afternoon snacks, you risk stacking them and breaking the 5 × 5 rule.

Remember that you don't have to count carbs for most of the lean protein, vegetable, or healthy fat choices (page 66). Only questionable foods (or those marked *) must be checked.

I have type 2 diabetes, take oral medication, and maintain a blood sugar of 200 mg/dL (11.1 mmol/L). Two weeks into Step One I find myself feeling a little shaky, dizzy, and sweaty, but when I check my blood sugar, it's normal—for the first time in years. Why am I feeling as if it's going too low?

Anyone with diabetes who takes medication to lower blood sugar (either oral or insulin) should inform his or her physician before beginning this program. Step One quickly improves blood sugar. Because your blood sugar has been out of control for a while, your brain has come to accept that 200 mg/dL as a normal reading, so the new "normal" level strikes your body as too low and you get all the symptoms of low blood sugar. As long as your blood sugar is in the normal range (over 70 mg/dL [3.9 mmol/L]), you do not need to treat it. Sit down, sip some water, relax, and the feeling will pass.

If you do not take medication for diabetes (oral medication or insulin), you will not become hypoglycemic on this program. If you are taking medication to reduce blood sugar and your blood sugar dips beneath 70 mg/dL (3.9 mmol/L), you have true hypoglycemia and must immediately treat the condition. Be sure to report low blood sugar readings ASAP to your doctor so that he or she may decrease the dosage of your medication and you can continue right along with Step One at a lesser medication dosage.

Can I eat as much as I want of the allowed foods on Step One?

Normal portion sizes of these foods are fine. For example, if you are hungry, there's no problem with having 8 ounces of lean protein at a meal. Huge portions, however, will thwart your weight loss. If you are hungry at any time, you can eat! Just make sure that the foods you choose are from the approved foods list and consumed in reasonable portions.

REAL READER SUCCESS STORY
Julie Wilson

Since October 2009, Julie has lost forty-three pounds.

Favorite MM Recipes: Chocolate Ricotta Pudding (page 315), Crustless Ham, Cheddar, and Veggie Quiche (page 220)

For most of her life, Julie reaped the benefits of hyperthyroidism, eating whatever she wanted without gaining an ounce of weight. However, as she got older, she began to suffer from fatigue, anxiety, and mood swings—and, despite working out three times a week and eating fewer calories, her weight kept climbing. In 2001 she was diagnosed with hypothyroidism. Medication didn't appear to be regulating her symptoms. In desperation, she looked to the Internet for answers. "I just typed in *metabolism* and the book popped up," she says. Julie followed the link to the book's Web site and discovered the Metabolism B checklist. She found herself saying yes to most of the symptoms. "I ordered the book and read the first chapter, and I couldn't believe it. It was like the author was talking to me!" she says.

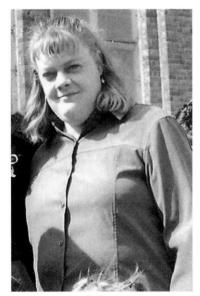

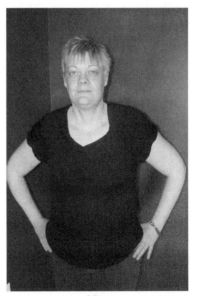

Before   After

The first four days were hardest for Julie. She had the shakes and felt nauseated as her body began to recover from the carbohydrate overload it had endured over the years. However, within two weeks, she noticed life-changing results: "Before, my doctors couldn't regulate my medication at all, but since I've been on Metabolism Miracle, my dosage has stayed the same."

Additionally, her sugar cravings disappeared and her energy shot up. "I used to sleep in the afternoons, and that stopped," she says. She began to feel calmer, and by the end of Step One, she had lost twenty-two pounds. "It was just a steady decline, and I've never put the weight back on," she says. "I find the plan very easy. You can eat a lot of food that I don't think you normally can on other programs. There's not a lot of weighing foods and not a lot of limitations."

Julie says that in the past, diets never worked for her: "I couldn't get rid of the sugar cravings, so I just gave up." But she didn't struggle with following the Metabolism Miracle program, and, even more impressively, she learned self-control. "I felt the program worked so well that I didn't want to sabotage what I was doing." she says. "Now I have a neighbor and a friend who are on it too because of what I've achieved."

Julie's biggest supporter in helping her reach her goal weight was her husband. He was careful to check in with her while grocery shopping and has started habitually reading food labels himself.

Recently, her family took a trip to the Caribbean. "I stepped out from behind my camera to be photographed, instead of trying to hide behind it," she says. "For once in years, I feel great about myself."

Julie's Advice

Make simple swaps for the foods you love. "I am a big chocoholic. I've gone from eating milk chocolate to 90 percent cacao, and that satisfies me."

6

STEP TWO—TRANSITION: A HEALTHY PATH TO CARBS

STEP TWO BASICS

TIME: 8 weeks or longer, until you reach your desired weight

CHALLENGE: Reintroduce healthy carbohydrates in the proper amount and at the right time, to promote continued fat burning and weight loss; gently restart your rested pancreas and liver

RESULT: Steady weight loss and continued improvements in blood sugar, cholesterol, triglycerides, blood pressure, and energy

During the eight weeks of Step One, you have lost fat inches and unwanted pounds. You no longer crave carbs, and you feel more energized than you have in years. You have completed your spring cleaning.

While you can feel and see the benefits of Step One, it helps to understand what internal changes have occurred to retune your metabolism. Your overactive pancreas has rested, and your liver has significantly decreased releasing glycogen. Your blood lipids (cholesterol and triglycerides) have markedly improved. Your fat cells have begun to shrink, and your insulin keys better fit the receptors on your cells. In short, your Metabolism B has

Before and After

Measure your progress in Steps Two and Three by stepping on the scale and taking your body measurements (chapter 10) only once a month. That way, you'll see dramatic changes without the erratic ups and downs of daily weight fluctuations.

been put in order so that it can behave normally. Step Two helps to reprogram it to process carbohydrates normally.

Now you are ready to reintroduce carbohydrates, the fuel that a healthy body needs to run properly. To do that, you must learn three key skills:

1. *How to introduce the mildest carbohydrates to a pancreas that has been resting for eight weeks*

2. *How to choose the right amount of carbohydrate at meals and snacks for continued weight loss and fat burn*

3. *How to place carbohydrate throughout the day—timing is everything!*

All of the foods that you ate freely in Step One you will continue to eat as base foods for Step Two. In addition, you will now add carb servings from a long list of low-impact carb foods. These foods will allow your pancreas to wake up slowly, preventing it from overreacting with excess insulin.

Step Two is a nutritionally balanced diet that allows safe, long-term weight loss. Plan to stay on this part of the program for at least eight weeks, until you have reached your desired weight. There is no limit to the amount of time you may stay on Step Two.

HOW IT WORKS

Let's take a look inside your body to understand exactly what happens when you reintroduce carbohydrates on Step Two. For the past eight weeks on Step One, your liver was intentionally depleted of glycogen stores so that it could not engage and cause blood sugar to rise and prod the pancreas into overreleasing insulin. Instead, both organs have rested. On the morning that you begin Step Two, the correct amount of low-impact carbohydrate will gently enter your bloodstream, and glycogen will once again be stored in the liver.

Once the liver has filled with glycogen, it is poised and ready to do its job. When you delay or skip a meal or fast during nighttime sleep, the liver goes into survival mode and releases a meal's worth of glycogen into your bloodstream. Every time your liver feeds you in this way, your pancreas overreleases the fat-gain hormone, insulin. The more often it happens, the more frazzled the pancreas becomes. Before you know it, your pancreas returns to

"But I'm Happy with Step One, and I Don't Want to Move On!"

After eight weeks on Step One, many patients tell me, "I never want to eat carbohydrate foods again. I look great, feel great, and my lab work is great. Why should I eat the food that caused all my problems?"

The cause of their problems was not carbohydrate. The cause stemmed from their Metabolism B overreacting to carbohydrate. Now that their system is back in balance, if they reintroduce carbohydrate the proper way, they will continue to lose weight and feel great.

My patients' carbohydrate phobia comes from their past experiences with other low-carb diets. When these programs reintroduce carbohydrate to the diet, low-impact carbohydrate is rarely emphasized. These diets offer no guidance on how much carbohydrate to introduce to the rested metabolism and when to schedule it into the day. Without proper guidelines regarding the introduction of carb, people with Metabolism B head right back to square one and experience rapid weight gain, low energy, and declining health.

As invigorating as Step One has proven for you, it is not healthy or normal to live on a very low-carb diet for longer than eight weeks at a time. *Very* low-carb phases are not nutritionally balanced, and eating this way for long periods of time will leave your pancreas and liver languid. Like every organ of the body, these two are designed to function. If they rest for too long, they may not perform efficiently when called upon in the future.

The Metabolism Miracle, in contrast to other low-carb diets, gives you very clear instructions on how to reintroduce carbohydrates the healthy way, continue to lose weight, and rediscover the joy in eating the many carbohydrate choices that fit this program.

overreleasing insulin, fat cells expand, insulin keys no longer fit the receptors, and hormonal imbalance returns.

Step Two is designed specifically to prevent the above scenario from occurring. By introducing a very specific amount of carbohydrate

(11–20 grams) no further than five hours apart, the liver will rarely be called upon to release glycogen. This proper reintroduction of carbohydrate minimizes the number of times per day that your liver engages. Consuming the correct amount of carb will also prevent the pancreas from overreacting to blood sugar rises from excess carbohydrate intake. You will take control of your blood sugar and prevent the pancreas from overreacting.

BACK TO THE TRUSTY FORMULA

So how do you keep your carbohydrates within the 11–20 gram range? You already know how to use the net carb formula because of the 5 × 5 rule in Step One.

Total carbohydrate grams—dietary fiber grams = net carb grams

In Step Two, you'll use the formula to guarantee that foods such as bread, crackers, cereal, bars, yogurt, and sugar-free ice cream stay within the 11–20 gram window. For example, you may want to eat a slice of whole-grain toast at breakfast. Whole-grain bread is mentioned on the Step Two "Low-Impact Carbs" list (page 92), but you'll want to make sure that the bread fits into the 11–20 gram allotment. Check the nutrition facts label and plug the numbers into your trusty formula.

SERVING SIZE: 1 Slice

TOTAL CARBOHYDRATE: 20 grams

DIETARY FIBER: 3 grams

20 – 3 = 17 net carb grams

This bread fits into the 11–20 gram window, so go ahead and enjoy it.

At lunch, you decide to have some multigrain crackers with your chicken Caesar salad. How many crackers can you have and still be within the 11–20 gram target range? Simply check the nutrition facts label.

SERVING SIZE: 8 crackers

TOTAL CARBOHYDRATE: 24 grams

DIETARY FIBER: 5 grams

24 – 5 = 19 net carb grams

Eight crackers fit into the 11–20 gram window, so go ahead and enjoy them.

For the next eight weeks, you should choose all of your carb servings from the "Low-Impact Carbs" list (page 92). The whole-grain bread and multigrain crackers are on the list. High-impact carbs such as marshmallows, potato chips, and fruit juice are not on the list. Keep them out of Step Two to prevent yourself from backsliding.

TIMING IS EVERYTHING

Once you enter Step Two, to keep your metabolism stoked, you must not exceed five hours without the inclusion of an 11–20 gram net carb food within every five-hour period, or else your liver will overcompensate with glycogen, you will stress the pancreas, and weight will come back. You'll have created the same metabolic monster that you transformed so successfully in Step One.

Remember that you are reprogramming your body. You want to program it with the right amount of low-impact carb at the right time. This is a period of transition. If you skip the transition and introduce carbs haphazardly, you will most definitely regain everything you've lost.

To recap: During Step Two, you must eat a food from the 11–20 gram net carb list at the following times:

- Prior to exercising if you exercise before breakfast

- With breakfast, lunch, and dinner

- At snacks between meals that are eaten more than five hours apart

- Right before you go to bed at night

- If you wake up during the middle of the night (an 11–20 gram snack is recommended but not required)

You have the option of having two "free" 5 × 5 carbs daily without adding their carb grams to your 11–20 carb "dam."

Choose all your 11–20 carb servings from the "Low-Impact Carbs" list (page 92).

What's Magical about 11 to 20 Carb Grams?

Once your liver is back from its vacation, the only way to control blood sugar response involves the timing and the amount of low-impact carb throughout your day.

Time your carbohydrates in the correct portions throughout the day, and you have effectively set up a dam that prevents the liver from releasing glycogen. It is critical to keep the amount of carbohydrate between 11 and 20 grams. A dam built of less than 11 grams will not be high enough to prevent liver glycogen from flowing over. A dam built of more than 20 grams of carbohydrate at a meal or snack will stimulate the pancreas to release extra insulin, and that will lead to weight gain rather than weight loss.

The easiest way to remember the details of Step Two is: Always place a carb dam (11–20 grams low-impact carb) to block the liver at:

Breakfast—within one hour of waking up
Lunch
Dinner
Bedtime snack—as close to bedtime as possible

If the time between breakfast and lunch will exceed five hours, you need to set a reinforcing dam with a midmorning snack (an additional 11–20 carb grams) to keep the liver on hold until you eat lunch. Similarly, if the time between lunch and dinner exceeds five hours, you will set a reinforcing dam with a midafternoon snack (an additional 11–20 grams) to stop the liver from spilling in the fifth hour.

On those days when you need to take the additional 11–20 grams as a between-meal snack, remember to also consume your 11–20 gram carb dam at the next meal. The 11–20 gram carb replacement at breakfast, lunch, dinner, and bedtime is a constant.

These 11 to 20 grams of low-impact carb, placed correctly, is what Step Two is all about. Proper placement enables the pancreas and liver to awaken gently and keep you in a weight-loss mode.

KEEP THEM COMING

It's hard to believe but, once you introduce carbs, you must keep them coming or you will regain weight. It is very possible that you'll need six or more carb servings per day.

Here's a typical day's carb placement for Step Two:

7:00 a.m.—Wake up

8:00 a.m.—Breakfast (11–20 g net carb)

11:00 a.m.—Midmorning snack with 11–20 g net carb (breakfast and lunch are greater than five hours apart)

1:30 p.m.—Lunch (11–20 g net carb)

4:30 p.m.—Midafternoon snack with 11–20 g net carb (lunch and dinner are greater than five hours apart)

7:30 p.m.—Dinner (11–20 g net carb)

10:30 p.m.—Bedtime snack (11–20 g net carb)

11:00 p.m.—Bedtime

(For specific examples, see "Step Two Sample Menu" on page 97.)

THE FIRST THREE DAYS OF STEP TWO

Most people notice that they feel a little bloated and their belts are a tad snugger during the first three days of Step Two. You are *not* gaining weight. As the liver refills with glycogen, it also takes in some additional fluid. Drink plenty of fluid during these days to help your body release the excess fluid. By the fourth day, the bloating will have disappeared and your waistband will be back to normal.

After those first three days, your body should continue to feel healthy and energized while you continue to lose weight. Learn Step Two as if it were your job. It will put you in control of your weight and health for life.

As with all of the steps of the Metabolism Miracle, be sure to follow the ten "Rules to Thrive By" (chapter 8). Pay particular attention to drinking at least 64 ounces of caffeine-free fluid daily, exercising a *minimum* of thirty minutes five times a week, and taking the recommended supplements.

Step Two is a nutritionally balanced, safe diet that you can follow for as long as you like and continue to lose weight. Once you have reached the weight that you desire and achieve maximum health on as little medication as possible, step on the scale and check your weight. The weight that makes you healthy and makes you look and feel great is *your* ideal body weight.

LOW-IMPACT CARBS

Choose any food from the low-impact carbs list for your breakfast, lunch, dinner, and bedtime snack. If the time between meals exceeds five hours, place an extra carb serving between them.

All portions shown are "ready to eat" and equal 11–20 grams net carb.

Breads

Read the label for breads, cereals, "bars," and crackers to make certain that dietary fiber is 2 grams or greater.

- 2 slices thin-sliced, light, or lower-carb whole-grain bread (2 g fiber or more)
- 1 slice whole-grain bread (2 g fiber or more)
- 1 light whole-grain English muffin (2 g fiber or more)
- ½ whole-grain English muffin (2 g fiber or more)
- 1 light or lower-carb whole-grain pita (2 g fiber or more)
- ½ whole-grain pita (2 g fiber or more)

5 × 5 Carbs

In addition to your necessary 11–20 gram net carb "dams," you may eat two 5 × 5 carbs on any day during Step Two (see "5 × 5 Carbs," page 53). You needn't add these carbs to the 11–20 gram total. Simply enjoy them as "free carbs."

Bread Tips

Fiber

When you buy breads, crackers, and cereals, make sure they have 2 grams or more of fiber, but don't trust the front packaging for that information. Always rely on the nutrition facts label. Grains that contain high amounts of dietary fiber take longer to digest and slow the glucose release into the bloodstream, making them perfect for people with Metabolism B.

Whole wheat bread generally has 2–3 grams of fiber per slice, a perfect choice for Step Two. In contrast, white bread, saltines, cornflakes, and many cereal bars have less than 1 gram of dietary fiber. They will cause blood sugar to spike and your pancreas to overreact.

Specialty Breads

Give thin-sliced, light, and lower-carb breads a try. With half the carbs of regular breads, they often allow you to have twice as much in your 11–20 grams net carb allotment.

1 slice of whole wheat bread = 2 slices of light whole wheat bread

Both of these bread choices have 2 grams of fiber or more and 11–20 grams net carb, making both choices perfect for Step Two.

Cereals and Grains

$\frac{1}{2}$ cup cooked oatmeal

$\frac{1}{2}$ cup cooked barley

$\frac{1}{2}$ cup cooked brown or wild rice

$\frac{1}{2}$ cup cooked whole-grain pasta (cook al dente)

$\frac{1}{2}$ cup cooked bulgur

1 serving dry cereal (2 g fiber or more)

Cereal for Breakfast?

When you want to eat cold cereal and milk for breakfast, remember that the combined milk and cereal net carbs must be 11–20 grams. A half cup of milk has 6 grams of net carb. Choose an unsweetened soy milk or low-carb milk as a free 5 × 5 carb, and you can have a larger portion of cereal.

Example:
¾ cup cereal = 9 g net carb
½ cup milk = 6 g net carb
Total: 15 g net carb

OR
1½ cups cereal = 18 g net carb
1 cup soy or low-carb milk = "free" 5 × 5 carb
Total: 18 grams total net carb (you can eat twice the amount of cereal!)

Crackers and Starchy Snacks

1 serving whole-grain crackers (11–20 g net carb and 2 g or more fiber)

3 cups popcorn (light or hot air–popped without partially hydrogenated oils)

1 serving whole-grain pretzels (11–20 g net carb and 2 g fiber or more)

1 serving tortilla chips (11–20 g net carb and 2 g fiber or more)

Protein Bars

Must contain 11–20 grams net carb and have 2 grams fiber or more.

Vegetables and Legumes

½ cup corn or ½ ear fresh corn

½ cup peas

½ cup legumes such as kidney beans, lentils, lima beans, chickpeas, white beans, black beans, or white kidney beans

½ whole or ½ cup mashed sweet potato or yam

1 cup raw or ½ cup cooked carrots

½ cup beets

Soups

1 cup tomato soup (water-based)

$\frac{1}{2}$ cup lentil soup

$\frac{1}{2}$ cup split pea soup

Fruit

All portions represent 11–20 grams net carb. Fruit choices should be average in size.

1 apple	12 cherries
1 pear	$\frac{1}{2}$ cup natural applesauce
1 peach	$\frac{1}{2}$ grapefruit (avoid if you are taking the medication Lipitor)
2 plums	
1 nectarine	1 cup whole strawberries (6–8 average-size berries)

Fruit Tips

Beware of Giant Fruit

When you choose fruit, take stock of its size. You needn't buy the smallest apple in the basket, but the orange that looks more like a basketball isn't a good option, either. Train your eye to focus on average-size fresh fruit that fits into the 11–20 gram net carb rule.

Just Say No to Juice

With its high-impact carbohydrate and negligible fiber, fruit juice spikes your blood sugar like a rocket, causing the pancreas of anyone with Metabolism B to overreact. Fruit juice is never a good choice if you have Metabolism B.

Missing Your Favorite Fruit?

If a preferred fruit is absent from the Step Two fruit category, it isn't an oversight. The fruits on this list are low impact and fit well into this transition stage when you are being cautious with your pancreas. Other fruits will come back into the picture when you enter Step Three.

³/₄ cup blackberries   8 dried apricot halves

³/₄ cup blueberries   12 grapes

1 cup raspberries   1 orange

2 clementine or 2 small   ³/₄ cup pineapple cubes
  tangerines   ¹/₂ banana

Milk and Other Dairy

1 cup (8 fluid ounces) milk (fat-free, nonfat, 1%, 2%, skim plus)

Plain yogurt (11–20 g net carb)

1 cup (8 fluid ounces) buttermilk (11–20 g net carb)

Fruit-flavored yogurt sweetened with Splenda or sucralose (11–20 g net carb)

¹/₂ cup sugar-free/fat-free pudding (11–20 g net carb)

No-sugar-added ice cream products sweetened with Splenda (11–20 g
  net carb)

Dairy Tips

How Low Can Your Milk Go?

Eight ounces of milk contain 11–20 grams of net carb, regardless of the milk's fat content. The benefit to using lower-fat versions is that they can help in a fat-burning weight-loss program.

Yogurt Choices

An 11–20 gram net carb light yogurt makes a great bedtime snack to keep your liver on hold and your pancreas in check. Don't confuse this light yogurt with the 5 x 5 version you had in Step One. Five grams of net carb is fine for an anytime snack, but it is not enough carb to "dam" your liver for the night ahead.

Welcome Back, Ice Cream!

Look for ice creams that have sucralose (brand name: Splenda) rather than sugar as the primary sweetener. Even if the net carb appears the same in sugar-sweetened ice cream, the type of carbohydrate is very different from that in Splenda-sweetened products. Sugar-sweetened desserts digest quickly with a high impact that spikes blood glucose.

STEP TWO SAMPLE MENU 1

Remember, timing is critical. You should never go more than five hours without an 11–20 gram net carb serving. In the sample menu below, each 11–20 gram net carb serving is noted, along with two "free" 5 × 5 carb servings.

6:30 a.m.—Wake up

7:00 a.m.—Breakfast

$1\frac{1}{2}$ cups cold cereal (11–20 g net carb) with 8 ounces low-carb milk (3 g carb, a "free" 5 × 5 carb)

Coffee with half-and-half and Splenda

10:00 a.m.—Midmorning snack

Handful of peanuts

You don't need an 11–20 gram net carb "dam" because breakfast and lunch are within five hours.

12:00 noon—Lunch

Grilled cheese sandwich made with 2 slices light whole-grain bread (11–20 g net carb)

Tomato wedges

Iced green tea

4:00 p.m.—Midafternoon snack

Dip of cottage cheese with 7 sliced strawberries (11–20 g net carb)

6:00 p.m.—Dinner

Broiled flounder

$\frac{1}{2}$ cup wild rice (11–20 g net carb)

Steamed broccoli

1 "Gilded" Cinnamon Muffin (recipe on page 313) (4 g net carb, second "free" 5 × 5 carb)

10:30 p.m.—Bedtime snack

1 serving peach-flavored light yogurt (11–20 g net carb)

STEP TWO SAMPLE MENU 2

6:00 a.m.—Pre-exercise snack

½ banana (11–20 g carb)

8:30 a.m.—Breakfast

4 ounces tomato juice (4 g net carb, first "free" 5 × 5 carb)

Egg substitute with 2 strips turkey bacon

1 light multigrain English muffin (11–20 g carb) with whipped butter

Coffee

Because breakfast and lunch are within five hours, you won't need a
  midmorning snack.

1:00 p.m.—Lunch

Scoop of tuna salad on a bed of romaine lettuce

15 thin wheat crackers (11–20 g net carb)

Flavored water

4:00 p.m.—Midafternoon snack

Part-skim string cheese and a handful of cashews

6:00 p.m.—Dinner

Roasted turkey breast with fat-free gravy

½ sweet potato (11–20 g net carb)

Green beans

Low-carb chocolate pudding (3 g net carb, second "free" 5 × 5 carb)

Sparkling water

11:00 p.m.—Bedtime snack

One ice-cream bar, sweetened with sucralose (11–20 g net carb)

STEP TWO SAMPLE MENUS
Breakfast Suggestions for Step Two

Miracle Quiche (recipe on page 219)

1 light multigrain English muffin (11–20 g net carb) with natural peanut butter and sugar-free jelly

Coffee, decaf, or tea with low-fat half-and-half and Splenda

Egg whites or egg substitute with ham and cheese

2 slices light whole-grain toast (11–20 g net carb) spread with whipped cream cheese

Coffee, decaf, or tea with low-fat half-and-half and Splenda

Grilled cheese: 2 slices light multigrain bread (11–20 g net carb), low-fat Cheddar cheese, tomato slices, and whipped butter

Coffee, decaf, or tea with low-fat half-and-half and Splenda

$3/4$ cup cereal with $1/2$ cup milk (11–20 g net carb)

Coffee, decaf, or tea with low-fat half-and-half and Splenda

$1\frac{1}{2}$ cups cereal with carb-controlled milk (11–20 g net carb)

Coffee, decaf, or tea with low-fat half-and-half and Splenda

$1/2$ cup cooked oatmeal or 1 prepared envelope unflavored cooked oatmeal (11–20 g net carb)

Sprinkle of cinnamon, walnuts, and Splenda

Coffee, decaf, or tea with low-fat half-and-half and Splenda

2 slices thin-sliced whole-grain toast (11–20 g net carb) spread with 1 teaspoon sugar-free jelly and 1 tablespoon natural peanut butter

1 cup carb-controlled milk (5 × 5 carb)

1 serving light yogurt or a light yogurt smoothie (11–20 g net carb), with walnuts added to yogurt

Zucchini Muffin (recipe on page 314) (5 × 5 carb)

Light cottage cheese

7 whole strawberries, sliced (11–20 g net carb)

Sprinkling of sliced almonds

"Gilded" Cinnamon Muffin (recipe on page 313) (5 × 5 carb)

1 light multigrain English muffin (11–20 g net carb) topped with egg whites or egg substitute, Canadian bacon, and whipped butter

Coffee, decaf, or tea with light half-and-half and Splenda

Lunch Suggestions for Step Two

Sandwich of 2 slices light whole-grain bread (11–20 g net carb), thinly sliced turkey breast, 1 slice low-fat cheese, lettuce and tomato slices, and light mayonnaise

Diet drink or flavored water

Cheesy Burger (recipe on page 264) on a light whole-grain burger bun (11–20 g net carb), with 1 tablespoon low-carb ketchup (5 × 5 carb), lettuce, tomato, and onion rings

Parmesan Chips (recipe on page 236)

Diet drink or water

1 low-carb pita (11–20 g net carb) filled with grilled chicken breast strips, shredded lettuce, shredded cheese, tomato wedges, and light dressing

Diet drink or flavored water

Chef's salad with cheese, turkey, ham, eggs, and light dressing

1 serving whole-grain crackers (11–20 g net carb)

Diet drink or flavored water

Easy Pizza (recipe on page 227); in place of the low-carb wrap from Step One, use a low-carb pita sliced in half to make 2 "pizza crusts" (11–20 g net carb)

Light cottage cheese

1 cup cubed melon (11–20 g net carb)

"Gilded" Cinnamon Muffin (recipe on page 313) (5 × 5 carb)

Diet drink or flavored water

1 serving light yogurt (11–20 g net carb)

Handful of almonds

Celery sticks with natural peanut butter

Tuna salad with light mayonnaise, on a bed of lettuce

Low-fat cheese cubes

Parmesan Chips (recipe on page 236)

½ cup Cold Pea Salad (recipe on page 249)

Diet drink or flavored water

Philly Steak and Cheese (recipe on page 279) on 1 light multigrain burger bun (11–20 g net carb) with sautéed peppers and onions

Cabbage Salad (recipe on page 245)

Sugar-free ice pop

1 cup tomato soup (11–20 g net carb)
Tender Spinach Salad (recipe on page 247)
Diet soda or flavored water

Chunky Chicken Salad (recipe on page 271) with vinaigrette dressing
$\frac{1}{2}$ cup Pasta Primavera Salad (recipe on page 250) (11–20 g net carb)
Diet soda or flavored water

Dinner Suggestions for Step Two

Roasted turkey with low-fat gravy
$\frac{1}{2}$ cup mashed sweet potato (11–20 g net carb)
French-cut green beans
Chocolate Ricotta Pudding (recipe on page 315)

Chicken breast
$\frac{1}{2}$ cup Pasta Primavera Salad (recipe on page 250) (11–20 g net carb)
Steamed spinach
Sugar-free gelatin with low-fat whipped cream

Grilled sirloin steak
8 Sweet Potato Fries (recipe page 309)
Tossed salad with light dressing
Chocolate Brownie Muffin (recipe on page 312) (5 × 5 carb)

Grilled 93% lean burger on 1 low-carb multigrain bun (11–20 g net carb)
    with light cheese, lettuce, tomato, light mayonnaise, and low-carb
    ketchup ("free" 5 × 5 carb)
Zucchini and Onions (recipe on page 308)

Chicken cheesesteak (with low-fat cheese) on 1 low-carb multigrain bun
    (11–20 grams net carb), with grilled peppers and onions and low-carb
    ketchup ("free" 5 × 5 carb)
Side salad with vinaigrette dressing

Miracle "Spaghetti" (recipe on page 275) with a sprinkle of Parmesan
    cheese and lean ground beef meatballs
2 slices low-carb multigrain "garlic bread" (11–20 g net carb)
Side salad with vinaigrette

Grilled pork chop
$\frac{1}{2}$ cup wild rice (11–20 g net carb)

Asparagus spears
Sugar-free gelatin with whipped topping

Chicken cutlet with low-carb bread crumbs (5 × 5 carb)
8 Sweet Potato Fries (recipe on page 309) (11–20 g net carb)
Broccoli spears
Sugar-free gelatin with whipped topping

Broiled flounder
Mashed Cauliflower (recipe on page 307)
Tender Spinach Salad (recipe on page 247)
Baked Apple (recipe on page 311)

Chicken Paprikash (recipe on page 266), served over ¹⁄₂ cup al dente
    whole-grain pasta (11–20 g net carb)
Sweet-and-Sour Cukes (recipe on page 247)
Cinnamon Ricotta Pudding (recipe on page 315)

Snack Suggestions for Step Two

Use these snacks only if an 11–20 gram net carb snack is required.
Whole-grain crackers (11–20 g net carb) with peanut butter or cheese
1 crisp apple with a dip of natural peanut butter
Baked Apple (recipe on page 311)
1 cup nonfat or 1% milk
1 serving light yogurt (11–20 g net carb)
1 protein bar (fiber over 2 g and 11–20 g net carb)
3 cups light popcorn (no trans fats) (11–20 g net carb)
¹⁄₂ cup light ice cream sweetened with Splenda (11–20 g net carb) and
    topped with nuts
³⁄₄ cup cereal with ¹⁄₂ cup 1% milk (total 11–20 g net carb)
1¹⁄₂ cups cereal with carb-controlled milk (total 11–20 g net carb)
¹⁄₂ cup sugar-free pudding cup (11–20 g net carb)
1 piece Step Two fresh fruit
1 serving whole-grain pretzels (11–20 g net carb)
¹⁄₂ cup natural applesauce
8 dried apricot halves and a handful of nuts
Sugar-free ice cream sweetened with Splenda (11–20 g net carb)

STEP TWO—FREQUENTLY ASKED QUESTIONS

How will I ever lose weight by adding carb to my diet?

With your Metabolism B, your weight is not entirely based on calories—it's based on the proper regulation of your blood sugar. Step Two strategically places a set amount of low-impact carb on top of a base of neutral foods so you can regulate your blood sugar. Without blood sugar peaks and valleys, your weight loss will continue.

My weight loss seems to have stalled on Step Two. Should I return to Step One?

During the first three days of Step Two, you might not lose weight because your liver will take on some fluid as it refills with glycogen. As long as you drink plenty of fluids during this time, you will lose the temporary water weight by day four.

Try not to obsess about pounds lost and focus instead on how you look and feel by the end of each step. The weight of people with Metabolism B will fluctuate on a day-to-day basis. Check your weight and body measurements the morning you begin Step 2 (see chapter 10), and don't measure again for at least one month. You will be pleased with your progress if you look at it over a period of time. Trust the program.

I'm confused by the five-hour rule. Is it a problem if I eat 11–20 grams of net carb in the morning and also three hours later? Won't I end up gaining weight because I've stacked carbs?

You must, without exception, eat 11–20 grams of net carb at breakfast, lunch, dinner, and bedtime. If your meals are closer than five hours and you add another 11–20 grams between them, they will stack and cause weight gain. Insert an 11–20 gram between-meal snack only if the meals are more than five hours apart.

I forgot to take an 11–20 gram snack when my meals were more than five hours apart. What now?

Every time you go longer than five hours without an 11–20 gram net carb dose, your liver releases a meal's worth of glycogen and your pancreas overresponds with insulin. As soon as you realize that you missed the five-hour mark, take the 11–20 gram carb allotment. Your liver doesn't dump the glycogen at one time; it continues until you put in the 11–20 gram allotment. If you realize that you've forgotten to take a "carb dam" between meals more than three times in a week, you need to return to Step One for a short ten-day detox to rest your metabolism. Then make a fresh start on Step Two.

I was sick for several days while on Step Two. Although I couldn't eat protein or vegetables, I made sure to eat my 11–20 net carb allotment. Is that enough?

That's perfect. If you have an unsettled stomach, use easily digested carbs such as 11–20 gram net carb crackers or yogurt, a half banana, or a half cup of natural applesauce in place of heavier carbs.

Now that I'm on a nutritionally balanced meal plan, should I continue to take my vitamins, minerals, and supplements?

Yes. Take them through all three steps of the Metabolism Miracle.

I'm constipated. What do you recommend for Step Two?

Do everything you would do during Step One—drink a minimum of 64 ounces of fluid daily, eat raw or al dente vegetables, increase your physical activity, and possibly use a plant fiber supplement. In addition, during Step Two, eat fresh fruit with skins intact, and make sure your grains contain at least 2 grams of fiber.

I love chocolate cookies, and two have only 16 grams of carb. Can I use them for an 11–20 gram net carb?

Not yet! Although those chocolate cookies contain the right *amount* of carb, the *type* of carb is wrong for the reprogramming phase. Cookies are sweetened with sugar and they lack the necessary 2 grams of fiber to fit the Step Two carb list. If you eat them, your blood sugar will spike and your pancreas will go into a hyper mode.

I can't seem to remember to take 11–20 gram net carb snacks between meals. Any suggestions?

Try using an alarm about four hours after the start of your last meal. Some people set an alarm on their computer or watch or use an actual pocket-size alarm. The alarm will remind you to decide if you will get your next meal within an hour. If not, you'll know to take a snack right then and there. Once it becomes part of your lifestyle to eat six times per day, you won't need the alarm. Routinely omitting your necessary between-meal snacks will cause weight gain and backsliding.

I have Metabolism B, but my husband, who also wants to lose weight, has Metabolism A. Can he use this diet plan for weight reduction?

Although anyone can follow the Metabolism Miracle program to lose weight, people with Metabolism B get a myriad of other rewards that are physical, emotional, and psychological. The Miracle is one of many weight-reduction plans your husband can follow, but it is the only weight-reduction and health-improvement plan designed especially for you.

I've asked my physician if alcohol is a problem, and she said that an occasional alcoholic beverage is allowed. Do I count the drink as 11–20 grams of net carbohydrate?

Although made from fruits and grains, the body does not process alcohol as a carbohydrate. Alcohol is processed like fat. If your physician has approved, you may drink alcohol—with the exception of regular beer, sweetened alcoholic beverages, cordials, liqueurs, and sweetened wines—on any step of the Miracle, but don't exceed two drinks, because the fat impact of alcohol will slow weight loss and fat burning. If you add a mixer, it must be water, seltzer, diet tonic, or diet soda rather than fruit juice or regular mixers.

REAL READER SUCCESS STORY
Gina Sheppard

Since July 2010, Gina has lost sixteen pounds.

Favorite MM Recipe: Silver Dollar Pancakes (page 225)

Gina's weight concerns began on the cusp of her fortieth birthday, when she was diagnosed with Crohn's Disease, a chronic digestive disorder. She lost more than thirty pounds within three months at the onset of the disease, but when she started treatment, she gained it all back—plus another 25 pounds. By October 2008, she was carrying 197 pounds on her five-foot-six-inch frame. Her waist size had inflated to forty-five inches, she was diagnosed with high blood pressure, and she frequently found herself feeling exhausted and mentally foggy. "I attributed it to Crohn's, medications, and all the things that make most middle-aged women tired, but my doctor couldn't explain it. I woke up tired and couldn't wait to go back to bed," she says.

Over the years, she tried dieting and swimming laps but struggled to get below 182 pounds. Although she regularly took fish and flaxseed oil supplements, ate salmon, and cut back on alcohol, she couldn't lose the belly fat or lower her triglycerides (high at 244).

In July 2010, Gina was waiting in the checkout line at the grocery store when she saw an article on MM that seemed to be speaking directly to her.

"Starting the plan was easier than I thought it was going to be," she says. "I was pretty skeptical about the whole thing at first, but I started feeling better immediately." The first person to notice a change was her mother, who declared how much more cheerful Gina had become. "I didn't notice the weight loss that quickly—it's been slow and steady," Gina says. "The thing that changed the most was my waist size," from which she dropped seven inches. "Knowing that is one of the worst places to gain, I was impressed."

One of Gina's hardest challenges was to avoid eating the breads, pastas, and rices that she used to have, but she's found some truly satisfying replacements: "I substitute tofu products for pasta, and I do cauliflower rice instead of regular rice; there are so many substitutions that I don't feel like I'm missing anything."

Though she's still in Step Two, Gina is proud to report that her triglycerides are now down to 103. Before she moves on to Step Three, her goal is a thirty-five-inch waist and whatever weight loss comes with it.

"I had given up, thinking I would feel crappy for the rest of my life, but this program has been life-changing for me," Gina says. "I have a lot more energy. I'm able to walk my dogs every single night—and these poor dogs had never been walked before!" She rejoices that she can get through the day without afternoon naps. Her Crohn's symptoms are under control, and finally, after years of illness and the side effects from medications, she says with relief, "I feel like I'm back to normal."

Gina's Advice

"Diane's blog really helped me a lot. She's on Facebook, and I can ask her questions. There really is someone there to help you."

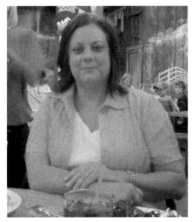
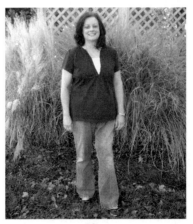

Before   After

7

STEP THREE—KEEPING
WEIGHT OFF FOR A
LIFETIME

STEP THREE BASICS

TIME: Lifetime weight maintenance

CHALLENGE: Opening your diet to more carbohydrates, including the treats that you may have been missing on Steps One and Two

RESULT: Keeping your health and energy levels in tip-top shape and maintaining your weight loss permanently

Congratulations! If you are beginning Step Three, you've reached the weight that makes you feel and look great. You've retuned your Metabolism B to handle carbohydrates properly and have given your body a brighter future.

As a maintenance phase that should last a lifetime, Step Three has two key benefits: a wider range of carbohydrate grams at meals and a wider variety of carbohydrate choices. While the low-impact carb choices from Step Two will always be preferable because they are high in fiber and nutritional value, the expanded carb list of Step Three will make occasional treats a possibility.

ONE STEP AT A TIME

Here's a recap of the three-step Metabolism Miracle.

Step One rested your weary metabolism by limiting net carbohydrates to 5 grams or less in a five-hour period (these were called "5 × 5 carbs"). You ate liberally of lean protein, heart-healthy fat, and neutral vegetables.

Step Two reprogrammed your rested metabolism and took you to optimal health and your desired weight. You ate 11–20 grams of low-impact net carbs at intervals of no greater than five hours. You ate liberally of lean protein, heart-healthy fat, and neutral vegetables and had the option of two "free" 5 × 5 carbs a day.

Now, with Step Three, you will maintain your newfound weight, health, and energy. You will identify the carbohydrate range that works best for your body, choose from an expanded variety of carb choices, and also have the option of two "free" 5 × 5 carbs a day. You will eat lean protein, heart-healthy fat, and neutral vegetables.

IDENTIFYING YOUR CARB RANGE

Now that you've reached your ideal weight, you will maintain that weight with a carbohydrate range that is specific to your individual body. In Step Two, you limited your net carbohydrates to 11–20 grams so that you could continue to lose weight. Step Three is less stringent, with a more generous daily carb allotment.

To identify a patient's ideal carbohydrate range, I use a classic nutrition formula that determines the number of calories a person needs to maintain his or her weight, neither gaining nor losing. Because a person with Metabolism B does not maintain weight solely by counting calories, I modified the classic formula to match the requirements of Metabolism B. When all the calculating is through, a person with Metabolism B will consume 30 to 35 percent of his or her calories from carbohydrate foods.

Activity Levels

Rate your activity level according to these three categories:

Sedentary = 30 minutes or less of physical activity 4 or 5 times per week
Moderate = 1 hour of physical activity 4 or 5 times per week
High = more than 1 hour of strenuous physical activity 4 or 5 times per week

You can quickly find your maximum number of daily carb servings to maintain your desired weight by pinpointing your sex, height, age, desired maintenance weight, and activity level on the following table. This is a very individualized way to determine carbs rather than a "one size fits all" chart. This easy method will allow both a six-foot-six, eighteen-year-old high school football player and his five-foot-one, seventy-year-old grandma to figure out the right amount of net carb for each of them.

CARB CHARTS

FEMALE 5′0″–5′3″
Maintenance weight of 100–130 pounds

AGE	ACTIVITY	MAXIMUM CARB SERVINGS/DAY
Teens	Sedentary	8.5
	Moderate	9
	High	9.5
20s and 30s	Sedentary	8
	Moderate	8.5
	High	9
40s and 50s	Sedentary	7.5
	Moderate	8
	High	8.5
60s and 70s	Sedentary	7
	Moderate	7.5
	High	8
80 and over	Sedentary	6.5
	Moderate	7
	High	7.5

FEMALE 5′4″ TO 5′7″
Maintenance weight of 120–150 pounds

AGE	ACTIVITY	MAXIMUM CARB SERVINGS/DAY
Teens	Sedentary	9.5
	Moderate	10
	High	10.5
20s and 30s	Sedentary	9
	Moderate	9.5
	High	10
40s and 50s	Sedentary	8.5
	Moderate	9
	High	9.5
60s and 70s	Sedentary	8
	Moderate	8.5
	High	9
80 and over	Sedentary	7.5
	Moderate	8
	High	8.5

FEMALE 5'8"–5'11"

Maintenance weight of 140–170 pounds

AGE	ACTIVITY	MAXIMUM CARB SERVINGS/DAY
Teens	Sedentary	10
	Moderate	11
	High	12
20s and 30s	Sedentary	9.5
	Moderate	10.5
	High	11.5
40s and 50s	Sedentary	9
	Moderate	10
	High	11
60s and 70s	Sedentary	8.5
	Moderate	9.5
	High	10.5
80 and over	Sedentary	8
	Moderate	9
	High	10

FEMALE 6'0"–6'3"

Maintenance weight of 155–185 pounds

AGE	ACTIVITY	MAXIMUM CARB SERVINGS/DAY
Teens	Sedentary	11
	Moderate	12
	High	13
20s and 30s	Sedentary	10.5
	Moderate	11.5
	High	12.5
40s and 50s	Sedentary	10
	Moderate	11
	High	12
60s and 70s	Sedentary	9.5
	Moderate	10.5
	High	11.5
80 and over	Sedentary	9
	Moderate	10
	High	11

MALE 5'0"–5'3"

Maintenance weight of 106–136 pounds

AGE	ACTIVITY	MAXIMUM CARB SERVINGS/DAY
Teens	Sedentary	9
	Moderate	10
	High	11
20s and 30s	Sedentary	8.5
	Moderate	9.5
	High	10.5
40s and 50s	Sedentary	8
	Moderate	9
	High	10
60s and 70s	Sedentary	7.5
	Moderate	8.5
	High	9.5
80 and over	Sedentary	7
	Moderate	8
	High	9

MALE 5'4"–5'7"

Maintenance weight of 130–160 pounds

AGE	ACTIVITY	MAXIMUM CARB SERVINGS/DAY
Teens	Sedentary	10
	Moderate	11
	High	12
20s and 30s	Sedentary	9.5
	Moderate	10.5
	High	11.5
40s and 50s	Sedentary	9
	Moderate	10
	High	11
60s and 70s	Sedentary	8.5
	Moderate	9.5
	High	10.5
80 and over	Sedentary	8
	Moderate	9
	High	10

MALE 5′8″–5′11″

Maintenance weight of 154–185 pounds

AGE	ACTIVITY	MAXIMUM CARB SERVINGS/DAY
Teens	Sedentary	11
	Moderate	12
	High	13
20s and 30s	Sedentary	10.5
	Moderate	11.5
	High	12.5
40s and 50s	Sedentary	10
	Moderate	11
	High	12
60s and 70s	Sedentary	9.5
	Moderate	10.5
	High	11.5
80 and over	Sedentary	9
	Moderate	10
	High	11

MALE 6′0″–6′3″

Maintenance weight of 178–210 pounds

AGE	ACTIVITY	MAXIMUM CARB SERVINGS/DAY
Teens	Sedentary	12
	Moderate	13
	High	14
20s and 30s	Sedentary	11.5
	Moderate	12.5
	High	13.5
40s and 50s	Sedentary	11
	Moderate	12
	High	13
60s and 70s	Sedentary	10.5
	Moderate	11.5
	High	12.5
80 and over	Sedentary	10
	Moderate	11
	High	12

MALE 6′3″–6′6″

Maintenance weight of 196–235 pounds

AGE	ACTIVITY	MAXIMUM CARB SERVINGS/DAY
Teens	Sedentary	13
	Moderate	14
	High	15
20s and 30s	Sedentary	12.5
	Moderate	13.5
	High	14.5
40s and 50s	Sedentary	12
	Moderate	13
	High	14
60s and 70s	Sedentary	11.5
	Moderate	12.5
	High	13.5
80 and over	Sedentary	11
	Moderate	12
	High	13

MALE OVER 6′6″

Maintenance weight of 226–250 pounds

AGE	ACTIVITY	MAXIMUM CARB SERVINGS/DAY
Teens	Sedentary	14
	Moderate	15
	High	16
20s and 30s	Sedentary	13.5
	Moderate	14.5
	High	15.5
40s and 50s	Sedentary	13
	Moderate	14
	High	15
60s and 70s	Sedentary	12.5
	Moderate	13.5
	High	14.5
80 and over	Sedentary	12
	Moderate	13
	High	14

One Size Does Not Fit All in the Family

Each member of this family has Metabolism B. But consider how the carbohydrate servings to maintain ideal weight vary for each person.

Dad: At forty-nine years old and a height of six foot three, Joe has reached his ideal weight of 210 pounds during the first two steps of the Miracle. He runs five mornings a week for one hour before heading off to work. On the "Carb Chart," a man of Joe's age, height, and moderate activity level needs *13 carb servings a day* to maintain his 210 pounds.

Mom: Sharon, also forty-nine years old and five foot five, has type 2 diabetes but got her blood sugar under control during Step One of the Miracle and felt great at 140 pounds by the end of Step Two. Sharon takes a brisk walk every evening for 45 minutes to an hour and takes the occasional bike ride on the weekend. On the "Carb Chart," a woman of Sharon's age, height, and moderate activity level needs *9 carb servings a day* to maintain her weight.

Daughter: As a student at graduate school, twenty-three-year-old Diana has maintained her ideal weight of 130 pounds for several years. She works out at a nearby fitness center four times a week for at least an hour. At five foot four, with her moderate activity level, Diana can eat up to *9.5 carb servings per day* without gaining weight. During exam week, when she can't find the time to get to the gym and her activity level enters the "sedentary" zone, Diana limits her carbs to 9 servings per day.

Son: Eighteen-year-old Phillip plays football on his high school team. Between practice and the games, he works out six days a week for more than two hours each time. According to the "Carb Chart," at six foot one and 220 pounds, a muscular teenager with Phillip's high activity level can eat up to *14 carb servings a day* without gaining weight. As he desires to maintain a slightly higher weight (muscle mass) during football season, he then adds 1 carb serving to the 14 he is allotted for his height/weight/activity and consumes 15 carb servings/day. During the off-season, Phillip still works out five days a week for at least forty-five minutes, but at this moderate activity level, he decreases his carb servings to 14 per day.

Now that you know the maximum number of carb servings that will maintain your ideal weight, take a look at the "Step Three Carbohydrates" list (page 000). You'll notice that all of the low-impact carb choices from Step Two show up on the list. But this time they're tallied in single-digit net carb servings rather than 11–20 gram net carb allotments. This makes Step Three easier for you to follow.

The key to Step Three is to spread your carb servings throughout the day. You'll still think in terms of five-hour intervals because that's how the liver works. And you'll have to be careful to get enough but not too many carb servings in any of those five-hour intervals. Eating too few carbs at a meal or snack allows the liver to kick in and release its glycogen stores. But eating too many carbs at a meal or snack will cause the rested pancreas to overreact. Both create havoc with Metabolism B and, ultimately, lead to weight gain.

To prevent such hiccups in Step Three, remember two simple rules:

1. *One carb serving is the minimum you may take at a meal or required snack.*

2. *Four carb servings are the maximum you may take at a meal.*

Although you must consume at least one carb serving at every meal or required snack, you needn't use your maximum carb servings on any given day.

Let's follow Sharon, the forty-nine-year-old mother with a maximum of nine carb servings per day. In her work as a health professional, Sharon

What Is a Carb "Serving"?

One serving of carb is any food with a net carb count of 11–20 grams. To make it easy, you can think of it as 15 grams on average. *In Step One,* you had to keep to the 5 × 5 rule and couldn't eat a full serving of carb.

In Step Two, you had to eat one carb serving (11–20 grams), making sure not to exceed five hours without an additional 11–20 gram carb snack.

In Step Three, you have great flexibility. The rule of thumb for carb servings in this phase is to spread your allotted carbs so that you have at least one carb serving at a meal or snack but no more than four servings at any time.

Most people like to think in terms of servings, but they know that each serving averages 15 grams. So four carb servings is equivalent to 60 grams of carb, and two carb servings is equivalent to 30 grams of carb.

is often rushed in the morning, has a quick lunch at her desk, takes an afternoon snack on the way to the gym, and has dinner at home. During the workweek, she distributes her maximum nine carb servings in this way:

6:30 a.m.—Wake up

7:00 a.m.—Breakfast: 2 carb servings

12:00 p.m.—Lunch: 2 carb servings

4:00 p.m.—Midafternoon snack: 1 carb serving

7:00 p.m.—Dinner: 2 or 3 carb servings

11:30 p.m.—Bedtime snack: 1 carb serving

Total carbs: 8 or 9

Following the basic rules, Sharon keeps her meals and nighttime snack to at least one and not more than four carb servings. When meals are more than five hours apart, the between-meal snack has at least one carb serving.

On the weekend, Sharon's schedule is quite different. She eats a pre-exercise snack in the early morning, enjoys a leisurely breakfast, a light lunch, and an afternoon snack; often eats dinner out; and has a light snack before bed.

Her carb placement for the weekend follows this schedule:

6:45 a.m.—Wake up

7:00 a.m.—Preexercise snack: 1 carb serving

9:30 a.m.—Breakfast: 2 carb servings

1:30 p.m.—Lunch: 1 carb serving

4:30 p.m.—Midafternoon snack: 1 carb serving

8:00 p.m.—Dinner: 3 carb servings

12:00 a.m.—Bedtime snack: 1 carb serving

Total carbs: 9

On a recent Monday, Sharon felt under the weather and spent the day at home, resting. She kept to the rule of at least one carb serving at every meal and snack but had no desire to eat her maximum nine carb servings. Instead, she ate one carb serving at all meals and snacks except dinner, when she ate two.

8:30 a.m.—Wake up

9:00 a.m.—Breakfast: 1 carb serving

1:00 p.m.—Lunch: 1 carb serving

4:30 p.m.—Midafternoon snack: 1 carb serving

7:00 p.m.—Dinner: 2 carb servings

10:00 p.m.—Bedtime snack: 1 carb serving

Total carbs: 6

Sharon's daughter Diana, who uses a maximum of 9.5 carb servings/day, normally takes two carb servings at breakfast and lunch and three at dinner. For snacks, she eats one to 1.5 carb servings. But because of an island vacation in two weeks, Diana takes her carb allotment down to a lower range . . . bikini season!

7:00 a.m.—Wake up

7:30 a.m.—Breakfast: 1 carb serving

12:00 p.m.—Lunch: 1 carb serving

4:00 p.m.—Midafternoon snack: 1 carb serving

7:00 p.m.—Dinner: 2 carb servings

11:00 p.m.—Bedtime snack: 1 carb serving

Total carbs: 6

In both cases, Diana also follows the rules, making no meal or snack less than one carb serving or greater than four. She has not exceeded her 9.5-gram allotment.

STEP THREE CARBOHYDRATES

All portions = 1 carb serving (11–20 g net carbs)

Breads

LOW IMPACT

2 slices light, thin-sliced whole-grain bread (2 g fiber or more)

1 slice whole-grain bread (2 g fiber or more)

1 light whole-grain English muffin (2 g fiber or more)

A Kitchen Scale

You may want to purchase a simple food scale for bakery bread, homemade bread or rolls, and bagels. Every ounce of bread is equal to one carb serving.

HIGH IMPACT

1 (1-ounce) slice white, whole wheat, rye, or pumpernickel bread

1 hot dog roll

1/2 burger bun

1/2 pita

3/4 ounce matzo

1 (1-ounce) chapati (use food scale)

1 (1-ounce) mini bagel or mini muffin

1/2 whole-grain English muffin (2 g fiber or more)

1 light or low-carb whole-grain pita (2 g fiber or more)

1/2 whole-grain pita (2 g fiber or more)

1 flour tortilla

1 soft taco shell

2 hard taco shells

1 frozen waffle

2 (4-inch) pancakes

Breading

1 (2–inch) cube cornbread

1 ounce bakery bread (use a food scale)

3/4 cup croutons

Cereals and Grains

LOW IMPACT

1/2 cup cooked oatmeal

1/2 cup cooked barley

1/2 cup cooked brown or wild rice

Bagel Bonanza

Bigger isn't always better. A mini bagel contains one carb serving, but the standard 4-ounce bagel most Americans eat packs four carb servings! Don't forget to count the breading on fish or chicken; on most items, it counts as one carb serving.

HIGH IMPACT

$\frac{1}{2}$ cup cooked cream of wheat

$\frac{1}{2}$ cup cooked farina

$\frac{1}{2}$ cup cooked grits

$\frac{1}{3}$ cup cooked white rice

$\frac{1}{2}$ cup basmati rice

$\frac{1}{2}$ cup cooked whole-grain pasta

$\frac{1}{2}$ cup cooked bulgur

$\frac{1}{3}$ cup cooked white pasta

$\frac{1}{2}$ cup pasta salad

$\frac{1}{2}$ cup macaroni and cheese

$\frac{1}{2}$ cup casserole dish made with pasta

Dry cereal plus milk = 11–20 g net carb (don't forget to combine carbs from both cereal and milk for the total amount)

Crackers and Starchy Snacks

LOW IMPACT

1 serving crackers with 2 g fiber or more = 11–20 g net carb inclusive (no trans fats)

3 cups popcorn (light or hot air–popped without partially hydrogenated oils)

1 serving whole-grain pretzels (11–20 g net carb and 2 g or more fiber)

1 serving tortilla chips (11–20 g net carb and 2 g or more fiber)

HIGH IMPACT

1 serving any kind of crackers containing 11–20 g net carb

1 serving chips with 11–20 g net carb

1 serving pretzels with 11–20 g net carb

$1\frac{1}{2}$ oblong graham crackers (3 squares)

Vegetables and Legumes

LOW IMPACT

$\frac{1}{2}$ cup corn or $\frac{1}{2}$ ear fresh corn

$\frac{1}{2}$ cup peas

$\frac{1}{2}$ cup legumes such as kidney beans, lentils, lima beans, chickpeas, white beans, black beans, or white kidney beans

$\frac{1}{3}$ cup hummus

HIGH IMPACT

$\frac{1}{2}$ cup mashed potatoes

$\frac{1}{2}$ baked white potato

3 ounces boiled potato

$\frac{1}{2}$ small order of french fries

Soups

LOW IMPACT

1 cup tomato soup (water-based)

$\frac{1}{2}$ cup lentil soup

4 slices melba toast

2 large rice cakes

8 small rice cakes

6 saltines

$\frac{1}{2}$ cup chow mein noodles

3 sandwich crackers with cheese or peanut butter filling

$\frac{1}{2}$ sweet potato or yam or $\frac{1}{2}$ cup mashed sweet potato or yam

$\frac{1}{2}$ cup cooked carrots or 1 cup raw carrots

$\frac{1}{2}$ cup beets

$\frac{1}{2}$ cup potato salad

$\frac{1}{3}$ cup baked beans

$\frac{1}{2}$ cup mashed plantain

1 cup winter squash

$\frac{1}{2}$ cup split pea soup

HIGH IMPACT

1 cup broth based soup with noodles, potatoes, rice, or barley

$\frac{1}{2}$ cup pasta e fagioli

1 cup "greens and beans"

$\frac{1}{2}$ cup minestrone soup

1 cup cream soup (high in fat)

1 cup chili with beans

Protein Bars

LOW IMPACT

Must contain 11–20 grams net carb and have 2 grams fiber or more

HIGH IMPACT

Any that contain 11–20 grams net carb

Fruit

All portions represent 11–20 grams net carb. Fruit choices should be average in size.

LOW IMPACT

1 apple	$\frac{3}{4}$ cup blackberries
1 pear	$\frac{3}{4}$ cup blueberries
1 peach	1 cup raspberries
2 plums	2 clementines or 2 small tangerines
1 nectarine	
12 cherries	8 dried apricot halves
$\frac{1}{2}$ cup natural applesauce	12 grapes
$\frac{1}{2}$ grapefruit (not allowed with Lipitor)	1 orange
	$\frac{3}{4}$ cup pineapple cubes
1 cup whole strawberries (6–8 average-size berries)	$\frac{1}{2}$ banana

HIGH IMPACT

4 rings dried apples	Dried fruit (11–20 g net carb serving size)
1 cup papaya cubes or $\frac{1}{2}$ papaya	
4 whole fresh apricots	1 kiwi
2 prunes	$\frac{3}{4}$ cup mandarin oranges
3 dates	1 cup watermelon, cantaloupe, or honeydew
2 tablespoons raisins	
2 figs	$\frac{1}{2}$ small mango or $\frac{1}{2}$ cup, chopped

Milk and Other Dairy

All portions represent 11–20 grams net carb.

LOW IMPACT

1 cup (8 fluid ounces) fat-free, 1%, or 2% milk

1 cup (8 fluid ounces) skim-plus milk

1 serving plain yogurt (11–20 g net carb)

$\frac{1}{2}$ cup sugar-free/fat-free pudding (11–20 g net carb)

HIGH IMPACT

$\frac{1}{2}$ cup ice cream (light, low-fat, regular)

1 serving fruit-flavored yogurt sweetened with sucralose or Splenda (11–20 g net carb)

No-sugar-added ice cream sweetened with Splenda (11– 20 g net carb)

$\frac{1}{2}$ cup frozen yogurt (light or regular)

Occasional Treats

These high-impact carbs are loaded with fat and have little nutritional benefit. Still, they can be a tasty treat from time to time. Each is listed in a typical serving size, along with its carb servings.

1 brownie, unfrosted (4-inch square): 2 carb servings

1 brownie, frosted (4-inch square): 4 carb servings

Cake, unfrosted (4-inch square): 2 carb servings

Cake, frosted (4-inch square): 4 carb servings

2 sandwich-type cookies with filling in the middle: 1 carb serving

2 cookies, average size, homemade, such as chocolate chip: 1 carb serving

1 frosted cupcake (small): 2 carb servings

1 plain cake doughnut: 2 carb servings

1 glazed-type doughnut: 2 carb servings

$\frac{1}{8}$ double-crusted fruit pie: 3 carb servings

$\frac{1}{8}$ single-crusted fruit pie: 2 carb servings

⅛ pumpkin or custard pie: 2 carb servings

⅛ large pizza: 3 carb servings

⅛ large pizza, thick outer edge of crust removed: 2 carb servings

1 bagel: 4 carb servings

½ bagel: 2 carb servings

1 hollowed-out bagel (insides scooped out): 2 carb servings

1 hard roll, kaiser roll, or 6-inch sub roll: 3 carb servings

1 hollowed-out hard roll, kaiser roll, or sub roll: 2 carb servings

1 wrap: 3 carb servings

1 cup of a casserole dish such as lasagna, mac and cheese, or tuna
   casserole: 2 carb servings

When You Can't Find a Food on the List

If you search for a food on the Carb List but you can't find it, there is another way
to determine its carb serving. Look on the nutrition facts label and convert the carb
grams to carb servings. Using the net carb formula (see page 56), first find the net
carbs, and then divide that number by 15 to find the "carb servings."

   For example:

POWER BAR

Serving size: 1 bar
Total carbohydrate: 46 grams
Dietary fiber: 8 grams
46 grams carb – 8 grams fiber =
38 net carb
38 ÷ 15 = 2.5
One power bar has 2.5 carb servings.

LARGE CHOCOLATE CHIP COOKIE

Serving size: 1 cookie
Total carbohydrate: 34 grams
Dietary fiber: 2 grams
34 grams carb – 2 grams fiber =
32 net carb
32 ÷ 15 = 2 (round off when close)
One cookie has 2 carb servings.

SOUP (1 CUP)

Serving size: = 1 cup
Total carbohydrate: 47 grams
Dietary fiber: 2 grams
47 grams carb – 2 grams fiber = 45 net carb
45 ÷ 15 = 3

Therefore, one cup soup has 3 carb servings.

Small fries: 2 carb servings

Medium fries: 3 carb servings

Large fries: 4 carb servings

1 breaded fish sandwich on a bun: 3 carb servings

1 breaded chicken sandwich on a bun: 3 carb servings

1 bun for large burgers or fast-food sandwiches: 3 carb servings

Sauce: 1 carb serving

1 cup Chinese rice, white or fried: 3 carb servings

6 chicken nuggets: 1 carb serving

6 pieces sushi: 1 carb serving

2 wontons: 1 carb serving

1 cup Chinese food such as beef and broccoli, or shrimp and veggies
    with sauce: 1 carb serving

Breading on any food: 1 carb serving

A DAY IN THE LIFE OF STEP THREE

Let's see how several more people handle the distribution of their
daily carbs.

Jeff's Step Three

Jeff is a thirty-three-year-old new father. Life is a little unsettled in the house
with a baby making demands, but Jeff wants to stay on the healthy road that
Steps One and Two have paved for him and keep up his hour at the gym four
times a week. At five foot ten, he wants to maintain 172 pounds. According to
the "Carb Chart," Jeff's allotment for maintenance is 11.5 carb servings per day.

Here's how Jeff spreads out those 11.5 carb servings.

5:45 a.m.—Wake up

6:00 a.m.—Breakfast: 2 carbs

Hollowed-out whole wheat bagel = 2 carb servings, with light cream
    cheese

Coffee with light cream and Splenda

9:30 a.m.—Midmorning snack: 1 carb

1 serving light yogurt = 1 carb serving

12:30 p.m.—Lunch: 2 carbs

2 slices whole wheat bread = 2 carb servings, with sliced turkey breast, Swiss cheese, lettuce, tomato, and a dab of mayo

4:40 p.m.—Midafternoon snack: 1 carb

Medium skim latte (using 8 ounces of milk) with Splenda = 1 carb

6:00 p.m.—Dinner: 3 carbs

Grilled chicken

Steamed broccoli

½ cup mashed potatoes = 1 carb

1 ear corn = 2 carbs

1 sugar-free ice pop (5 × 5 carb, as it contains 3 grams net carb)

10:00 p.m.—Bedtime snack: 1 carb

1 light multigrain English muffin = 1 carb, spread with natural peanut butter

3:00 a.m.—Feeding for the baby . . . and Jeff!

8 ounces nonfat milk = 1 carb

Carb Servings Made Easy

If you'd rather avoid doing the math to determine carb servings from carb grams, tuck this cheat sheet into your wallet for an easy reference. Once you know the net grams of a food, you can find that number on this chart, and the conversion of net carb grams to carb servings is done for you.

IF YOUR NET CARBS ARE . . . THEN YOUR CARB SERVINGS ARE . . .

5.5–10 gram range = 0.5 carb serving

11–20 gram range = 1 carb serving

21–25 gram range = 1.5 carb serving

26–35 gram range = 2 carb servings

36–40 gram range = 2.5 carb servings

41–50 gram range = 3 carb servings

51–55 gram range = 3.5 carb servings

56–65 gram range = 4 carb serving

More than 65 grams of carb = *Too much!*

Nadine's Step Three

Nadine works in an office all day and takes thirty-minute walks four times a week at lunch with a work buddy. At fifty-two years old, Nadine enjoys her sedentary lifestyle but would like to maintain her 128-pound weight on her five-foot-three frame. According to the "Carb Chart," Nadine's allotment is 7.5 carb servings.

Here's how Nadine chooses to spread her 7.5 carb servings.

6:45 a.m.—Wake up

6:00 a.m.—Breakfast: 2 carbs

> 2 slices thin-sliced whole wheat toast = 2 carb servings, with whipped butter
> Egg whites
> Herbal tea

10:30 a.m.—Midmorning snack: 1 carb serving

> 1 peach = 1 carb serving
> Handful of almonds

1:00 p.m.—Lunch: 1 carb serving

> 1 low-carb wrap = 5 grams net carb ("free" 5 × 5 carb) filled with tuna salad made with light mayonnaise plus lettuce and tomato
> 1 (1-ounce) bag baked chips (17 grams net carb) = 1 carb serving
> Diet soda

4:30 p.m.—Midafternoon snack: 1 carb serving

> 1 serving light yogurt = 1 carb serving

7:00 p.m.—Dinner: 2 carb servings

> 5 ounces wine (with MD's okay)
> Grilled tilapia
> Large garden salad with balsamic vinaigrette
> Broccoli spears
> Baked potato = 2 carb servings, with whipped butter or light sour cream
> Sugar-free gelatin dessert

11:00 p.m.—Bedtime snack: 1 carb serving

> 7 strawberries with light whipped cream = 1 carb serving

IF YOU BEGIN TO GAIN WEIGHT

The ease and flexibility of Step Three allows you to vary your carb intake within your maximum range and have tremendous freedom with your carb choices. Meanwhile, lean protein, heart-healthy fat, and neutral vegetables continue to be unlimited, and you can still use two "free" 5 × 5 carbs per day. Maintaining your weight is an indication that you are eating a very reasonable amount of protein, fat, and veggies and getting adequate physical activity.

If, despite staying within your carb targets, your weight begins to creep up, you need to take a moment to analyze the situation. There are only a handful of reasons that would cause your weight to increase:

- You've exceeded your maximum carb servings.

- You've eaten less than 11 grams of net carb at a meal or snack.

- You've let five hours go by without a minimum of one carb serving.

- You are heavily overeating proteins and fats.

- You aren't getting thirty minutes of exercise five times a week.

- You're suffering increased stress, a recent illness, or increased pain.

The easiest way to determine why your weight might be creeping up is to keep a detailed three-day food diary that includes the timing of meals and snacks, the foods chosen, and how much of the food you've eaten. You should also note how much and how often you exercise and whether you have suffered any stress, pain, or illness of late.

When you review your three-day food diary, ask yourself:

_____ Are my portion sizes of carb foods correct?

_____ Are there gaps of over five hours without a carb serving?

_____ Did I forget to take a carb serving within an hour of wakeup?

_____ Did I skip a carb serving before bed?

_____ Am I overeating noncarb foods?

_____ Did I exercise adequately?

DAILY FOOD LOG

Time	Food Eaten with Amount

Stress Level Today:
_____ Low
_____ Medium
_____ High

Exercise Today:
_____ Minutes

Decaffeinated Fluid/
Water Today:
_____ Ounces

Vitamins/Minerals
Today:
_____ Yes
_____ No

_____ Am I unusually stressed?

_____ Am I in pain?

_____ Am I feeling ill?

It's easy to fix forgotten carb servings or to cut down on excessive portions of noncarb foods. As for exercise, it's a matter of making up your mind and getting back into your routine. But stress, pain, and sickness are often out of your control and can result in hormonal shifts that cause increases in blood sugar, pancreatic activity, and ultimately, weight.

You may not be able to control the source of stress, but you may be able to diminish the physical toll it takes on your body. Many people successfully use yoga, deep-breathing techniques, or positive visualization. Others pump up their physical activity to counter increased stress hormones. Work with your physician to help minimize chronic pain. One school of thought maintains that waiting too long to treat pain causes additional problems. This line of thinking supports treating pain before it gets a grip on physical and mental health.

Illness triggers the release of stress hormones that are needed for the self-healing process. Unfortunately, these hormones cause a natural rise in blood sugar that causes the pancreas to overrelease insulin, the catalyst of weight gain. Take care of yourself with rest, proper nutrition, vitamin/mineral supplementation, fluids, and physical activity to lower your risk of weight regain.

THREE STRIKES, YOU'RE OUT

Think of the above causes of weight gain as "strikes." I teach my patients the "Three-Strike Rule." If you look over your log and find that in a one-week period, you've upset the pancreas three or more times, you've struck out and need to send your pancreas to a short stint in detox, back to Step One.

Unlike people with Metabolism A, who can just restart their diet when they stray off course, those with Metabolism B must start with a clean slate. Return to Step One for ten days, during which your pancreas and liver will rest. Then progress to Step Two for ten days to reprogram your metabolism. After ten days you may either continue with Step Two or move on to Step Three.

A QUICK MENTION OF "SLIPUPS"

You're bound to have a few slipups as you live the MM lifestyle. Twice a year—during the winter holidays and also during my summer vacation—I intentionally relax my program. After these breaks, I reset my metabolism with ten days of Step One followed by ten days of Step Two. For more on slipups, see Chapter 8.

STEP THREE—FREQUENTLY ASKED QUESTIONS

The bottom line with Step Three is that I can eat more carbs, yes?

Yes. Designed for lifetime weight maintenance, Step Three offers an expanded range of carbohydrate. The lower end of the range remains at one carb serving (11–20 grams). The upper end of the range is unique to your situation but should not exceed 65 grams (four carb servings).

If I decide that I don't want more than one serving of carb per meal or snack, can I live on this amount of carbohydrate over the long term?

You can. If you begin to lose weight beyond your ideal weight, increase your intake of lean protein and heart-healthy fats.

Does it benefit me to keep my carbohydrate intake near the lower end of the range?

Any carbohydrate amount within your maintenance range is perfectly fine. You needn't deprive yourself by staying to one carb serving per meal when you desire two or three. Just be sure not to exceed your maximum servings per day.

My jeans are getting snug in the waist. What's the quickest way to return to my comfortable, healthy size?

Weight gain for people with Metabolism B is not usually a function of excess calories; it is a function of excess weight-gain hormones and **lack of exercise**. Create a three-day food diary and identify what might be causing the fat gain (see page 126). Once you have found the culprit, you will need to detox with ten days on Step One to reprogram your body, followed by ten days on Step Two, and then work to avoid this situation in the future.

Now that I'm on the maintenance portion of my plan for life, should I continue taking supplements and drinking green tea?

I wish I could tell you that you can get all of your needed vitamins, minerals, and antioxidants from the foods you regularly consume. In my opinion, however, because our food supply is overprocessed and tinkered with chemically and hormonally, we may be missing out on some of what we need. I think of the Miracle's supplements and green tea as insurance to make certain that my body gets what it requires.

Can I ever ease back into a "normal" lifestyle, or will I be forever timing my meals, counting carbs, and reading food labels?

The Metabolism Miracle is the "normal" way of life for your body. If you eat haphazardly, your pancreas will overreact with excess insulin, you will regain weight, and you will begin to experience all the symptoms that fluctuating blood sugar once caused—fatigue, depression, anxiety, restless sleep, midline fat, blurry vision, irritability, and carb cravings. In time, you could develop type 2 diabetes and require daily medication.

Don't think of the Metabolism Miracle as a quick fix or just another weight-loss program. It is the healthiest lifestyle for a person born with your metabolism. It will keep you at your healthy weight and size on the least amount of medication.

I have two children who seem to be manifesting Metabolism B. My daughter is ten and my son is fifteen. Is it wise for them to begin the program now?

Growing children require a balanced diet for growth and increased energy demands. I'm reluctant to start young children on the Metabolism Miracle program because Step One is not a balanced diet. I rarely recommend the program for boys until they have reached the age of eighteen, when much of their growth is complete, or for girls until at least two years after the start of their first menstrual period.

If, however, their pediatrician analyzes their blood with a metabolic panel, thyroid panel, lipid panel, and HbA1C and finds that their numbers point to Metabolism B, I would not hesitate to put a child on four weeks of Step One followed by Step Two, until healthy weight and labs are attained. They can follow Step Three for life with no problem whatsoever.

Your child's pediatrician should help with determining healthy weight, and a registered dietitian can figure out a healthy carb allotment of 30 to 35 percent, using a pediatric calorie formula.

If their labs are normal and they are too young to begin the entire Metabolism Miracle program, you can still teach them healthy eating patterns:

- Start each day with a breakfast that includes lean protein and is not too high in carbohydrate content. Think scrambled eggs with half the yolks removed, a light multigrain English muffin, half banana, and a glass of skim milk.

- Encourage healthy lower-carb snacks between meals, such as natural peanut butter, low-fat cheese sticks, low-carb yogurt, or lean turkey roll-ups.

- Get them into the habit of a snack before bed that includes lean protein and perhaps a high-fiber starch, such as peanut butter on whole wheat toast with a glass of skim milk.

- Limit high-impact carb snacks, including white flour crackers, potato chips, white flour pretzels, cookies, and candy.

- Eliminate fruit juice from your home. Let your children get their fruit requirement from a piece of fresh fruit instead.

- Avoid giving children and teenagers artificial sweeteners and caffeine. Consider using half the sugar in a recipe.

REAL READER SUCCESS STORY
Diana Kresefski

Since June 2004, Diana has lost twenty-nine pounds.

Favorite MM Recipes: Chocolate Brownie Muffins (page 312), Pasta-Free Veggie Lasagna (page 290)

Perhaps no one one, other than the author herself, has been eating the Metabolism Miracle way as long as her daughter, Diana. Her troubles began at age seventeen. She had been active her whole life, participating in soccer, softball, and competitive cheerleading. All of a sudden, without changing her diet or her intense level of activity, she began to grow a belly, love handles, back fat, and a chubby face.

"No matter what I did—no matter how much I exercised or how little I ate—I gained weight and was soon the biggest one out of all my friends," Diana says. She was always exhausted, could no longer focus in school, and soon started having anxiety attacks, which came more and more frequently the longer she struggled with her weight and the resulting depression. "Something was happening to me, and I didn't understand it until I began the Metabolism Miracle lifestyle," she says.

Diana learned that because all four of her grandparents, as well as her mother, had type 2 diabetes, she had a genetic predisposition to Metabolism B.

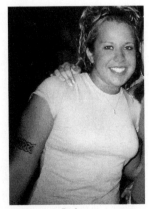

Before

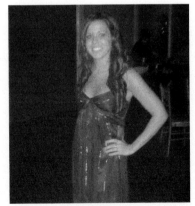

After

"I'm lucky enough that my mom is Diane. She never pushed it on me, but it got to the point where she said, 'You need to feel good; just try it,'" Diana says. Among other changes, she started switching out her breakfast toaster pastries and cereal bars for egg whites with ham or turkey bacon. Within two days of starting the plan, Diana saw changes in her energy levels. She could focus better in school and, as she continued Step One, her anxiety attacks disappeared.

"It felt like a cloud had been lifted off," she says. "Soon the excess bloat receded, and my love handles went away." By the end of Step One, Diana was wearing medium tops and size 9 pants. She stayed on Step Two until she got down to her goal weight of 126 pounds. Now on Step Three, she has kept off her 29-pound weight loss permanently since 2005.

"Nobody really knew I was dieting, so when I first lost the weight, people were shocked," Diana remembers. "I guess people assume that when you lose a lot of weight, you gain it back. But I didn't. Not only that, but I have always maintained the great way I feel—emotionally, physically, and mentally. I learned that I have the power to change how I feel, and I didn't need pills to do it. I no longer need to take antianxiety medication (the only medication I was on), and my period has been regular every month since beginning this amazing lifestyle program. I'm proactive about my health now instead of backtracking to fix it later in life."

Diana's Advice

You can do this. "It's not just a diet. It's not a short-term quick fix. It's a lifestyle change, and it's designed to fit into your lifestyle."

8

RULES TO THRIVE BY

As you follow all three steps of the Metabolism Miracle, keep the ten easy "Rules to Thrive By" in mind. Before you know it, they'll be such a part of your life that you won't even have to think about them.

RULES TO THRIVE BY

1. *Drink at least 64 ounces of water and other caffeine-free fluids.*

2. *Avoid gaps of more than five hours without a meal or snack.* Spread your food intake throughout the entire day and even into the night. Within one hour of waking up and right before bed, be sure to have a meal or snack.

3. *Take the recommended vitamins, minerals, and supplements.*

4. *Choose nonnutritive sweeteners with care.* I recommend the use of sucralose or stevia as a sugar substitute.

5. *Judge the carbohydrate content of packaged foods by reading the nutrition facts on food labels and using the net carb formula (see "Easy Carb Counting," page 55).*

6. *Consider drinking green tea daily.*

7. *Increase your physical activity to include a minimum of thirty minutes five times per week.*

8. *Eat allowed foods liberally but not to excess.*

9. *Practice relaxing.* Take a few minutes each day to close your eyes, breathe deeply, shed your stress, and clear your mind.

10. *Think positively!* First thing in the morning and the last thing at night, remind yourself of your good health, weight loss, high energy level, continuing progress, and positive future.

Most of the rules have already been explained in earlier chapters. This chapter will give you more information on why you need to drink at least a half gallon of fluid every day, why you need to spread your food throughout the day, why you should consider drinking green tea, and which supplements you should consider.

DRINK UP!

When you're on a fat-burning regimen, it is absolutely critical that you drink enough fluids. Fat burning leaves waste products that must be cleared from the bloodstream. Without enough fluid, your blood becomes overly concentrated with waste products. The brain senses this and borrows fluid from your tissues to dilute the blood. The brain then intentionally slows down fat burning until the blood is properly diluted. As you can see, it's vitally important to drink enough fluids on a fat-burning program or you will in fact slow your weight loss. I recommend drinking at least 64 ounces (a half gallon) of caffeine-free fluid each day.

Two Quick Ways to Check Hydration

Don't judge your need to drink water by your thirst. After the age of twenty, the body's ability to sense dehydration gradually begins to diminish. By age seventy, there can be little to no warning of your hydration status.

To gauge whether you're drinking enough, use the following two methods.

1. *When urine is deep yellow in color, it may be overly concentrated.* Check the color of your urine. If you are drinking enough fluids, it should be pale yellow in color.

2. *Here's an unscientific but trusty indication of your fluid status.* Put one hand, palm side down, on a table. Pinch together a little skin from the top of your resting hand and hold the pinch for a count of five. Let the skin go and

see how long it takes for the pinched skin to return to normal. A hydrated hand will smooth out quickly; an underhydrated hand will return to normal slowly.

Fluids containing caffeine do not count in the 64-ounce allotment because caffeine acts as a diuretic that causes you to eliminate more fluid than you have taken in. When you drink 12 ounces of coffee, you will urinate more than 12 ounces. This leaves you less hydrated than before you drank the coffee! For this reason, I don't recommend more than two caffeinated beverages per day during Steps One and Two of the Metabolism Miracle.

Green Tea

Much of the hubbub in the news about green tea comes from an antioxidant in the leaves that is released when the tea is steeped. The antioxidant EGCG (epigallocatechin gallate) contained in green tea leaves has been linked to a reduced risk of breast, prostate, colon, and skin cancers; the lowering of LDL cholesterol and aiding in the breakdown of fat; the prevention of dental cavities; and blood thinning.

I recommend a minimum of two green tea bags per day (most advocates consume at least four bags per day). Steep one or two tea bags into a cup of boiling water for more than three minutes. Consume the tea on the same day it is brewed, to ensure its potency. Decaffeinated green tea seems to have less potency than caffeinated green tea.

Get your green tea the old-fashioned way, by steeping it in boiling water. Bottled green tea beverages rarely contain active EGCG, nor have green tea extracts, concentrates, or pills shown the benefits of steeped green tea.

Green Tea: Caffeine with Benefits

Consider counting green tea as one of your two caffeine-containing beverages. A cup of tea made from two green tea bags steeped in one cup of boiling water contains about the same amount of caffeine as a cup of coffee but with tremendous antioxidant benefits!

What Beverages Should You Consume?

Pure water should make up the majority of your fluid intake. To keep track, consider drinking your water from bottles or a half-gallon pitcher. Four 16-ounce water bottles contain 64 ounces. When I am at the office, I place my empty water bottles under my desk. It may look a little messy, but at the end of the workday, I count the bottles and know how much additional fluid I should drink during the evening.

Other good choices include:

- Flavored water

- Flavored or plain seltzer

- Some fitness waters (check label for net carb)

- Caffeine-free and herbal tea

- Decaffeinated coffee

- Caffeine-free diet soda

- Club soda

You May Need More Than 64

Not everyone gets enough mileage out of 64 fluid ounces. A large-framed man might need more; a small-framed woman may need less. In any case, drink, drink, and drink. It's a great way to care for yourself and one of the easiest things you can do to protect your health.

If constipation plagues you, take extra precautions to drink enough fluid. The majority of patients I see who complain of constipation do not drink enough throughout the day.

EAT ALL DAY LONG

A popular diet program allots dieters a certain number of points that relate to the number of calories they may use in the course of the day. According to this plan, as long as their point allotment is used up at the end of the day, the dieters are on course. Another famous diet plan cautions dieters to "avoid eating after 6:00 p.m.!" because evening calories go straight to fat. These popular theories work *against* anyone with Metabolism B. Your weight is not based on the textbook formula:

Calories eaten – calories burned off during exercise = weight

With Metabolism B, you must spread your food out throughout the entire day. Eat within one hour of waking up, don't let more than five hours pass without a meal or snack, and end your night with a snack right before bed. Anytime you block the liver from releasing glycogen, you have better control of your blood glucose, insulin release, and fat deposits. You truly do have to eat to lose weight!

When more than five hours pass without eating, your body automatically lowers its metabolic rate. Alternatively, by spreading meals and snacks throughout the day, your body stays in a more awake metabolic rate that burns consistently higher. Think of eating all day as though you were putting kindling on a fire. If you dump it all on the flames initially, the fire will burn brightly but will burn out quickly. When you instead fuel the fire with kindling throughout the day and night, the fire will burn steadily. Food is the kindling for Metabolism B. Eating all day gives the most steady, long-term burn.

Get in the habit of eating throughout the entire day on Step One to make the practice second nature for the rest of your life.

VITAMINS, MINERALS, AND SUPPLEMENTS

The following supplements help to optimize health at any time, but they are particularly important during Step One of the Metabolism Miracle, when you are temporarily restricting certain foods. They have all been shown to work well with the Metabolism Miracle's goals—long-term fat loss, higher energy, and improved health. Inform your physician of any supplements you intend to take, and carry in your wallet at all times a list of the medications and supplements that you take.

Multivitamin with Minerals Supplement

Dosage: One daily multivitamin with minerals supplement

This supplement provides insurance that you will meet the recommended daily intake of vitamins and minerals. Women of childbearing age should choose a multivitamin/mineral that contains iron to help replace iron lost during menstruation. Men can choose a formula designed specifically for men. Women past menopause can use formulas designed specifically for older adults, as they no longer lose blood on a monthly basis.

Calcium

Dosage: 500–600 mg taken twice a day

Calcium is needed for more than bone strength, from heart regulation to hormone secretion. If you fail to ingest adequate calcium through diet or supplements, your body will leech calcium from your bones and teeth, leading to decreased bone density and possibly osteoporosis.

Purchase calcium that has been combined with vitamin D and magnesium for improved absorption. Calcium comes in different forms, including calcium carbonate, which must be taken with food, and calcium citrate, which can be taken without food. If you regularly take antacids, choose calcium citrate. Because the human body can absorb only 600 milligrams of calcium at one time, split your daily dose by taking a maximum of 600 milligrams of calcium at one meal and the other 600 milligrams of calcium at another. If calcium supplements constipate you, drink more water. You might also start with half the full dosage for the first week and increase your dosage the following week.

Fish Oil (Capsules)*

Dosage: 1,000–2,400 mg per day

Fish oil or omega-3 fatty acids help to reduce coronary vascular disease by decreasing triglycerides and blood pressure, decreasing the growth of

---

* Consult with your physician before beginning omega-3 supplementation, especially if you have a low platelet level or take a blood thinner such as warfarin (Coumadin). Excessive intakes may cause bleeding.

atherosclerotic plaque, and decreasing the stickiness of blood platelets, therefore helping to thin the blood.

I recommend 1,200 milligrams per day for heart-healthy people and 2,400 milligrams per day for anyone with heart disease. It's also a good idea to eat fatty fish, such as sardines, albacore tuna, mackerel, and salmon, twice a week. These fish contain high amounts of two kinds of omega-3 fatty acids: EPA (eicosapentaenoic acid) and DHA (docosahexaenoic acid).

Vitamin E*

Dosage: 400 IU (d-alpha tocopherol)

Vitamin E has been linked to a decrease in coronary vascular disease and helps to stop damage to cell membranes from free radicals. Because vitamin E is fat soluble, you can't excrete excesses through urine, so before taking vitamin E, look at the amount already contained in your multivitamin/mineral supplement. Together, the two supplements shouldn't exceed the recommended 400 IU.

The natural version of vitamin E, d-alpha tocopherol, is more active than the synthetic form. Check your vitamin E label for the lowercase *d* to make sure you choose the right form.

* Check with your physician before beginning vitamin E supplementation.

When Should You Take Your Supplements?

Divide your supplements, and take them on a full stomach at two different meals in the day for optimum effectiveness, as follows:

MEAL 1	MEAL 2
• 1 multivitamin with minerals	• 400 IU vitamin E
• 500–600 mg calcium with magnesium and vitamin D_3	• 500–600 mg calcium with magnesium and vitamin D_3
• 1,000–1,200 mg fish oil	• 1,000–1,200 mg fish oil
• 1 B-complex vitamin (B-50)	

SLIPUPS: BREAKS TO HELP STAY THE COURSE

The Metabolism Miracle is designed to help you reach and maintain permanent weight loss, improved health, and overall well-being. In a balanced life, there will be special times such as holiday meals, celebrations, vacations, and social gatherings, when you make the decision to go off your plan for a meal or a brief time. These little breaks can be very helpful in staying the course. I always plan to slip up on my birthday dinner, my anniversary celebration, certain food-related holidays, and vacation. These are planned slips, and I know exactly how to accommodate them without jeopardizing all the positive things I've accomplished.

On the Metabolism Miracle program, those slipups generally fall into two categories.

1. *The party or special occasion slipup:* When most dieters plan a celebratory meal, they usually save up calories during the day and indulge at the party. One popular weight-loss program uses a point system, allotting points to be saved up and placed anywhere in the day. You are now well aware that this system can never work with your body's physiology because your weight is a function not of calories but of the overprocessing of blood sugar into fat cells.

With the Metabolism Miracle program, if you want to go off your plan for a celebratory meal, don't change anything during that day to compensate for the party. Leave your day exactly as it should be up until the party meal, enjoy the party, and then return to your plan that night with the appropriate snack. Metabolism B does not allow you to make up for a slipup by changing an earlier or later meal to have less carbs.

Enjoy your slipup meal and then return to your plan. I don't recommend allowing yourself a slipup more than once a week.

A Sample "Party" Day

7:00 a.m.—Breakfast (with appropriate carb target)

10:30 a.m.—Midmorning snack (with appropriate carb target)

1:00 p.m.—Lunch (with appropriate carb target)

4:00 p.m.—Midafternoon snack (with appropriate carb target)

6:30 p.m.—Party (you're not counting carbs)

11:00 p.m.—Bedtime snack (with appropriate carb target)

2. *The long weekend, holiday, or vacation slipup:* For a typical dieter, it's the excess calories that cause weight gain during a vacation or holiday. For anyone with Metabolism B, it's the extra carb, lack of carb, timing of carb, and/or type of carb. Vacation shakes up your routine, and that means meals may get delayed without snacks, you may sleep late, or you may eat foods whose carbs are higher than you thought.

On vacation, too many or too few carbohydrate servings cause blood glucose to rise and the pancreas to wind like a top. The best way to handle these extended slipups is to reprogram your system once you're home again. As soon as possible upon returning home, start a quick ten-day detox, using the guidelines for Step One, followed by ten days of reprogramming with Step Two. It's quite easy this time around:

Detox: Ten days of Step One

Reprogram: Ten days of Step Two

Back to Basics: Return to Step Two or Three, whichever you were on prior to your vacation

I sometimes consider eating out at an unconventional restaurant as a planned slipup. This way, I can order sensibly from the menu without fretting that the carb probably exceeds my target range. Remember to stay within your carb range right up to and after the "out of the ordinary" meal. Don't try to make up for excess carbs.

Never fret after a planned slipup of several days. Remember that *The Metabolism Miracle* is written for you, and you are meant to lead a full and healthful life. You now know how to occasionally accommodate a little food "fun" without negative repercussions. The trick is to plan for the slipup as well as for the cleanup afterward. Move forward in a positive direction, don't wallow in guilt, and get back on track so you can continue to reap all the benefits of your new and improved life.

You'll soon know the "Rules to Thrive By" so well that they'll simply become a part of your life, just as a child learns the ABCs. Follow these guidelines to help you keep yourself healthy and energized.

The Healing Powers of Peppermint

Breath freshener, appetite suppressant, and digestive aid, too? Having some peppermint in the form of a Lifesaver, two Altoids, or a cup of tea (brew dried leaves, or try peppermint green tea) can be a very beneficial after-meal habit!

REAL READER SUCCESS STORY
Merrilee Felix

Since December 2009, Merrilee has lost fifty-five pounds.

Favorite MM Recipes: Chicken Paprikash (page 266), Seafood Delight (page 288)

"I've been overweight from the time I was little," says Merrilee, a sixty-three-year-old retiree. She went on her first carbohydrate-restricted diet at age fourteen, but she was never able to stick to a diet plan: "As soon as I would quit, the weight would come back, plus more—always."

In addition to being overweight, she suffered from chronic depression as well as chronic diarrhea that had stuck with her since she had her gallbladder removed at age twenty-five. When she was then diagnosed as prediabetic, something in her snapped.

"I was at a stage in 2009 where I just sat down and said a prayer to God," she says. "I said, 'Lord, if this is not the way I should be, then show me.' It wasn't two weeks later that I was standing in the grocery line with all my carbohydrates and all my junk food, and there was an issue of *First* magazine there. I read about the Metabolism Miracle and thought about it and thought about it. I finally bought the book and started reading, and I bawled. It was like this book had been written just for me: 'Dear Merrilee, here's your wake-up call.'"

Unlike the other plans she had tried—only to quit five days later—Merrilee found the Metabolism Miracle to be simple. She made a commitment to follow it and learned what to look for and what to watch. "The methodology around Metabolism Miracle made more sense to me than the information I was given by my dietitian at the diabetes class I went to," she says.

According to Merrilee, everything about this plan has indeed been a miracle for her. Her blood sugars were balanced within four months of starting the plan, and her doctor reduced her diabetes medications. Within ten months, she was completely off the medicine, and her blood sugar has stayed between 80 and 96 every day. Merrilee has shed nearly sixty inches total from her body and has gone from wearing size 3X and 4X styles down to XL tops and size 14 pants.

She's still working on flattening her tummy, but she's thrilled with her results so far: "It's so amazing to be able to feel my ribs, hip bones, and thighbones," says the five-foot-one woman. "As I get closer to my goal weight of 150, I start to think I can get to 135."

Merrilee was forced to retire early at the age of fifty-one because of her long-term chronic diarrhea, but those symptoms finally stopped when she went on the eating plan. Her chronic depression let up, too: "I'm a survivor and I always have been. The depression got better because I felt better about myself."

During retirement, Merrilee accumulated many sedentary hobbies, such as painting, crocheting, and doing puzzles. These creative outlets

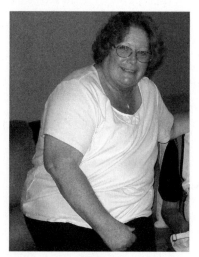
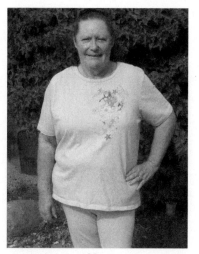

Before   After

helped her cope with her health issues but didn't lead to positive physical results.

"Exercise is so important, and I don't believe I realized that until I did this plan," she says. Now she lifts weights for her arms, rides her bike for three miles three days a week, swims laps, and is trying to master the hula hoop. "As a person who never did exercise, I have more fun now than I've had in years," she says. "It's not a chore like it was before."

Merrilee's Advice

"I read the MM board every day. Everyone has such interesting stories! We keep everyone updated on the foods that we eat daily. I'm so amazed at how creative everyone is, especially with the swaps they make to stay on Step One."

9

THE CRITICAL LINK: EXERCISE

Y ou don't need a gym membership, expensive equipment, or a personal trainer for the exercise piece of the Metabolism Miracle. All you need is a minimum of thirty minutes a day.

Throughout years of counseling patients in weight loss, I've found that people are more willing to make dietary changes than to add exercise to their life, regardless of how important exercise is to the weight-loss equation. They get exhausted thinking about workouts even before they attempt to do them. That's because most exercise programs are based on burning calories; they stress aerobic activity with a warm-up, a workout at target heart rate, and a cool-down. This type of program is often impractical, repetitious, and unrealistic. As a result, many exercise programs start off with a bang and end up as a memory.

Keep in mind that in the case of Metabolism B, your weight is *not* entirely the result of eating more calories than you burn. Your weight is mainly a function of hormonal imbalance.

Doctor Approval

If you haven't been exercising regularly, consult with your physician prior to beginning. He or she may need to review your medications, check your blood pressure, do an orthopedic exam, or perform an EKG or exercise stress test. All of those reviews will help determine the best type, duration, and intensity of your workout.

Exercise stimulates muscle cells to burn more blood glucose. This results in a lesser release of insulin. Exercise is a "nonmedicine" medicine for fat loss. In addition, physical activity tones your muscles and helps direct your body to focus on burning fat. It perks up your metabolic rate, improves mood, and helps relieve stress.

MAKE IT BURN

Your goal is to burn fat and maintain muscle. If you've been sitting around for the past week, doing little more than walking from your house to the car and from the parking lot to your office, then your muscle has been relatively inactive.

Imagine that your fat tissue and *inactive* muscle tissue appear dark blue. The brain cannot distinguish between the two and chooses either when it needs fuel to burn for energy.

When you get off the couch for an evening walk, that exercise causes the muscle tissue to activate. Think of it as changing from dark blue to bright red. The brain can now clearly distinguish between the two and will choose to consume the fat tissue, leaving the muscle intact.

Muscle is metabolically active tissue. Once stimulated, it burns calories for hours after the workout. The more muscle tissue a body has, the more furnaces it has and the more efficiently it handles food. Fat's main functions, on the other hand, are to insulate the body and to provide a stockpile of calories for times of famine. Fat is not metabolically active and does not burn calories at rest.

As long as you have exercised in tandem with the Metabolism Miracle diet, your brain can clearly differentiate between muscle and fat tissue—and will choose to burn the fat. If, however, you decide to remain sedentary, the brain will burn both fat and muscle tissue. You will lose weight, but, along with the fat you hoped to lose, you also lose valuable muscle.

LESS IS MORE

I once had a patient with Metabolism B who followed the Miracle program with his wife. He exercised faithfully for thirty minutes five times a week, but she opted not to exercise. When they returned in eight weeks for a follow-up, the wife had lost more weight on the scale than her husband, but she felt a little weak and tired. Oddly, he looked as if he had lost far more weight than his spouse. He had trimmed five inches off his waist, looked slimmer, and felt more energized. In addition, his lab work showed impressive decreases in cholesterol, triglycerides, glucose, and blood pressure.

As she gloated about her greater weight loss, I had to explain that without exercise, her brain had been directing her body to burn both muscle and fat tissue.

Muscle, being the heavier tissue, showed up as more weight loss. But in fact, this woman had lost valuable furnaces for burning fat. Her husband, who burned only fat tissue, which is fluffy and voluminous, looked as if he had lost significantly more.

Leona, the Frustrated Exerciser

Leona, a vice president of a successful business firm, had a stubborn roll of fat around her middle and felt out of shape, fatigued, and older than her forty-six years. With her tight schedule, Leona wanted to get the most bang for her efforts and see results quickly. She hired a personal trainer to tailor a program specific to her needs.

The trainer started her on a five-day workout program with a mix of exercises, including cardio, weight training, and body sculpting. Leona took the regimen seriously, determined to whip her body into shape.

Several weeks passed and the scale did not budge. The trainer explained that because muscle tissue weighs more than fat tissue, she might not immediately see weight loss, as heavy muscle tissue was replacing lighter fat. Leona could live with that theory if her body looked different. But despite the intense workouts, her paunch stayed put, as if a layer of fat covered her muscle. There was no sign of toned, sculpted muscles even as the weeks turned into months.

Eventually, the trainer, who did not quite believe Leona was being honest about her diet, referred her to my office for evaluation, saying, "It is impossible for Leona to eat the amount of foods that she reports, to work out to the degree she does, and have no significant results."

HOW MUCH AND WHAT KIND OF EXERCISE DO YOU NEED?

To retain muscle tissue and burn fat tissue, you need to increase your physical activity over your own personal norm. You will need a minimum of thirty minutes of increased activity for a minimum of five days per week.

If your daily routine contains built-in activity, like that of a waiter, construction worker, nurse, or mother of twin toddlers, your body has come to expect this level of daily activity. This is your norm. You'll have to add thirty minutes of activity to your day for the muscle activation that the Miracle requires.

Some Metabolism B dieters wonder if, instead of five days at thirty minutes, they can do two and a half hours of exercise in one day out of the week. It's a nice concept, but your muscle tissues need regular stimulation so that your brain will target fat cells on a daily basis. One day of activity will burn fat for that day but will not direct the brain for the next day. Move your

Leona had fasting blood glucose of 98 mg/dL ([5.4 mmol/L]; normal in the Miracle program is 65–89 mg/dL [3.6 mmol/L–4.9 mmol/L), and the doctor had flagged her LDL cholesterol and triglycerides as high. She walked into my office looking forlorn and said, "You are my last hope. I am watching everything I eat, counting every calorie and fat gram, exercising my backside off, and I can't lose inches or pounds." Sure enough, her food log showed that she was eating the calories of a woman who weighed forty pounds less. She began checking off the symptoms for Metabolism B. She was fatigued, depressed, and irritable. She had midline fat and carb cravings and had recently suffered her first panic attack. Her mother had type 2 diabetes.

Within a few weeks of starting the Miracle program, Leona began to see the difference in her body. She kept up a weekly routine at the gym, but this time, as she burned fat, her muscles showed tone and form. She also lost weight for the first time in months. Even better, she regained her energy and felt brighter and calmer.

By her next physical exam, Leona's lab work had returned to normal. She has remained on the maintenance phase of the Metabolism Miracle for over four years and says, "It's not a diet, it's my way of life."

muscles throughout the course of the week and your brain will consistently choose to burn fat tissue.

The type of physical activity that you choose is up to you. Mix it up to stimulate different muscle groups and to keep your interest. Walking, swimming, gardening, biking, yoga, light weight lifting, weight training, skiing, snow shoveling, tennis, using elliptical machines, aerobic exercise, and swimming all stimulate muscle tissue (see "21 Easy Ways to Start Moving," page 151.)

If your mobility is restricted, check with your physician about armchair exercises that might work for you, such as the use of light hand weights while watching television. If you pick up a two-pound weight and lift it during commercials, putting it down when the program returns and shifting arms for the next batch of commercials, you can easily activate muscle tissue for thirty minutes without leaving your chair during the course of a two-hour television movie.

As your body acclimates to exercise, add a few more minutes on the treadmill, a few more pounds of weight, or a few more sit-ups. Some people leave the thirty minutes intact but increase the pace. Each subtle change reinvigorates the body and keeps your exercise out of the norm for your body. Dance to another song or walk an extra block. Never stagnate—always move forward.

SCHEDULE EXERCISE AROUND YOUR MEALS

The timing of exercise makes a difference for people with Metabolism B. You will benefit the most if you schedule it around meals and snacks. These simple guidelines will maximize your fat burning by complementing your metabolic system.

If you work out first thing in the morning, eat a preexercise snack. As you already know, when you first awaken, your body is running on glycogen that the liver has released after five hours without food. If you exercise without eating, your liver will continue to release sugar throughout your routine. That will stimulate your pancreas to release much more insulin than it would release if you ate a light snack. Excess insulin will open more fat cells and cause fat gain. You could be exercising in the morning and gaining weight!

For the most efficient workout, exercise one to two hours after the start of a meal. Your blood glucose hits a peak one to two hours after you begin to eat. If you time your activity for this peak period, the muscles you activate during

21 Easy Ways to Start Moving

1. Take a brisk ten-minute walk before work, a fifteen-minute walk at lunch, and a ten-minute walk before you go home.

2. During two hours of television programming, instead of munching through the thirty minutes of commercials, lift hand weights, do calisthenics, or climb the stairs several times.

3. Work in your garden.

4. Mow your lawn (with a walking mower).

5. Take a yoga class.

6. Clean out the garage.

7. Wash the floors the old-fashioned way.

8. Wash your car by hand.

9. Ride your bike or walk to get the morning paper or go to the post office.

10. Work out to a thirty-minute exercise video.

11. Take an after-dinner walk with your family or a brisk walk at the mall with a friend.

12. Pace the sidelines during your child's athletic games, or walk the track before the game begins.

13. Bike to the park and back.

14. Swim, play tennis, or play golf (without the golf cart).

15. Take a hike.

16. Walk your dog.

17. Take the stairs instead of the elevator.

18. Play tag, jump rope, and try the hula hoop or scooter with your children for at least thirty minutes a day.

19. While on a conference call, walk throughout the conversation or lift light weights at your desk.

20. Turn on your favorite music and dance.

21. Wear a pedometer and compete with a friend to see who walks the most steps per day over a month's time.

your exercise session will use sugar from the food and allow much less insulin release and fat storage.

Take a snack before exercising if it's been four or more hours since you've eaten. If four or more hours have gone by since you last ate, it is best to take a preexercise snack. That way you won't cross into the five-hour mark without realizing it.

KEEPING TRACK OF YOUR TRACKS

Keep a log of your exercise in a prominent place, such as the refrigerator door. It will help you see your progress and remind you when you need to set aside thirty minutes for more activity.

Use the chart below to start your record. When you complete thirty minutes, put a check in the box. If you add extra minutes, jot them next to the "thirty minutes" check. Five check marks are needed per week minimally.

Treat the squares on this chart like the sections of a pillbox. You wouldn't skip taking your blood pressure medication, so don't skip taking your exercise. It's the critical link for anyone on the Miracle program.

FREQUENTLY ASKED QUESTIONS ABOUT EXERCISE

I don't have a thirty-minute block of time in which to exercise. Is it worth doing less?

You don't have to exercise for thirty minutes in succession. The idea is to energize your muscles for at least thirty minutes above and beyond your normal level of activity. It's fine to get your exercise in intervals: fifteen minutes or more in the morning, fifteen minutes or more in the evening. You can even consider ten-minute intervals three times a day.

I want to lose as much weight as possible. If I can skip the exercise and lose more weight, I'm going to skip the exercise.

Stop! It's true that if you were to follow the diet regimen of the Miracle without exercising, you would lose more weight on the scale. But you would lose valuable muscle along with your fat, and, ultimately, that's not the weight loss you want.

After day three of Step One, your brain must choose to burn either fat or muscle tissue. Daily exercise steers your brain to choose fat, which is big and fluffy and makes you look particularly heavy. When you don't exercise, your body will also choose to burn muscle, the heavy dense tissue that gives you firmness, shape, and tone.

Keep in mind that muscle cells are like little furnaces that burn fat even when you are asleep. When you exercise, you will save the muscle and burn the fat. So please exercise.

I've heard that to get any health benefit from exercise, I must have a warm-up, at least thirty minutes of cardio, and then a cool-down. Your program is much easier. Will I really get a workout and lose weight with this program?

The answer depends on what you want to achieve. It takes at least thirty minutes of aerobic activity at your target heart rate to begin to attain cardio benefits. Weight lifting helps tone muscle and maintain bone mass and fits the Miracle requirement of thirty minutes a day five times a week. But weight lifting doesn't get your heart rate into the cardio zone. Gardening requires muscle stimulation and also fits the Miracle requirement but probably won't get you to the cardio level. Running for thirty minutes achieves both.

Each of the activities mentioned above stimulates muscle so that the body will burn fat instead of muscle tissue. If you want a cardio workout as well, make sure that thirty minutes of your workout contain aerobic activity, such as walking, jogging, and swimming.

I cannot imagine eating a snack before I exercise in the morning. I want to burn this excess fat, not the food I'm eating before I walk!

As a person with Metabolism B, when you follow Steps Two and Three, you will use food as a way to stabilize your blood sugar and minimize insulin release. The small snack you eat before exercising will stop your liver from overreleasing sugar stores and stimulating the pancreas to overrelease insulin and open more fat cells. The snack blocks weight gain and enhances weight loss.

I understand the need to block the liver while I'm exercising. What if I exercise two or three hours after a meal? Do I still need that preexercise snack?

Fueling Intense Exercise on Step One

Take this advice on Step One for exercise that lasts more than forty minutes and is of a moderate to high level of intensity.

The first eight weeks of the Metabolism Miracle is a "means to an end" phase that's necessary to allow the pancreas and liver to rest and rehabilitate. For the organs to rest, the carbohydrate content must be low enough to keep the glycogen stores in the liver and muscles emptied. This temporary low-carb step definitely accommodates regular exercise, such as forty minutes of walking, weight training, swimming, or gardening. For moderate- to high-intensity exercise that lasts longer than forty minutes, your body will require an additional fuel source. This "fueling forward" enables you to have a great workout without "hitting a wall" or becoming exhausted. Fueling forward will energize your workout. After you finish exercising, you'll be back to normal, with no leftover carb effects!

Choose one of the following for each ½ hour of activity: an apple, an orange, ½ banana, ½ cup natural applesauce, 8 ounces Gatorade, four glucose tablets, or 1 tablespoon honey.

1. At the start of the workout that will exceed forty minutes, choose one serving from above list. This will fuel your first ½ hour of activity.

2. After ½ hour is complete, take another single serving from above. This will fuel the upcoming ½ hour.

3. Repeat as above for each upcoming ½ hour of exercise.

Then take one of the following protein choices within thirty minutes of completing your workout: a low-carb shake (with 2 grams or less net carb grams), one piece of string cheese, a spoonful of natural peanut butter, or your next Step One meal or snack.

"Fueling it forward" ensures that the athlete in training will have enough fuel to take him/her through the workout and have the blood sugar back to normal afterward.

If you have eaten less than four hours before you exercise, you won't need to take a snack. If you are going to begin exercising four hours or more after you've eaten, take an appropriate snack.

Examples:

6:00 p.m.—Dinner

8:00 p.m.—Exercise requires no snack

6:00 p.m.—Dinner

10:00 p.m.—Exercise does require a snack

I like to bike two hours after breakfast. If the ride lasts two hours, should I snack afterward so as not to go too long between meals?

Absolutely. Try never to go more than five hours between meals, regardless of whether you are active during that time. You will feel better if you eat an 11–20 gram snack after your ride to stop the liver from releasing at hour five.

MONTHLY EXERCISE LOG

MONTH_____

	MONDAY	TUESDAY	WEDNESDAY	THURSDAY	FRIDAY	SATURDAY	SUNDAY	DAYS/WEEK
Week One								
Week Two								
Week Three								
Week Four								

Put a check in the box if you've exercised at least 30 minutes that day.

REAL READER SUCCESS STORY
Larry Sayette

Since March 2010, Larry has lost twenty-four pounds.

"I was always a gym rat and thought I was healthy," says Larry, an automotive salesman from New Jersey. "I was strong in the gym, and that was how I judged myself. What a mistake."

After his son was born in January 2010, Larry applied for a better life insurance policy. "I received the results of the requisite physical exam with both shock and dismay," he says. "Not only was my cholesterol in the stratosphere, but my liver enzymes and insulin levels were incredibly high."

Larry immediately scheduled an appointment with his doctor, who confirmed the insurance exam results. "I don't see you getting out of this without medication," his doctor told him. But Larry wouldn't settle for medication. "I'm a believer that the body can heal itself if you put it in the right environment," Larry says. He told his doctor he would see a nutritionist.

That nutritionist was Diane Kress. She warned Larry that he was dangerously close to a stroke. He had seen firsthand how the Metabolism Miracle could yield dramatic changes. After the birth of their daughter five years earlier, his wife had tried the eating plan and lost forty pounds.

Getting started on Step One was hard, especially the first four days, but Larry says that by the end of that period, several amazing things happened: "My allergies went away. I mean *gone*. I just woke up on the fourth day and I could breathe. My energy levels were at hyper levels too, which surprised me, since I used to crash at 3:00 p.m. without fail."

After ten days, he noticed his weight dropping: "I was melting. It was almost like time-lapse photography. From day to day I could see the difference."

The plan has helped Larry change both his eating habits and his gym routine. He was always a real meat-and-potatoes guy, but now he swaps out potatoes for vegetables like asparagus. "I'll make a sauce with mustard, mayo, sea salt, and garlic," he says. "It's this thick, rich sauce that tastes amazing, and I don't have to worry about the carbs." He admits that before starting the Metabolism Miracle, he was never big on vegetables, but "now I go out of my way to eat broccoli and string beans."

As he lost weight, his power in the gym went down, too, so he altered his routine to incorporate lighter weights and more cardio. "I used to train like a lifter, not like a runner, and now the doctor says I have the numbers of a professional athlete," he says. In less than a year, his heart attack risk dropped from a score of 9.9 (out of 10) to 2.7. His blood pressure is down to 110/68, his cholesterol plummeted from over 300 down to 128, and his resting heart rate is sitting pretty at 54 beats per minute.

"If I hadn't lost the weight, I think I would have stroked out," he says. He recently turned fifty and has nothing but good health to show for it. "I look younger, and I have more energy. After seeing me, my boss and coworkers went out to get the book!"

Larry's Advice

On the road to maintenance, it's okay to take a step backward. "I've been able to maintain my weight on Step Three, but if I'm getting headaches or feeling tired, I'll go back to Step Two."

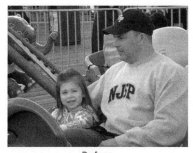

Before

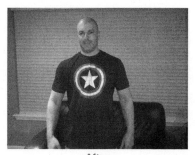

After

10

MEASURING UP: HOW TO MONITOR PROGRESS WITHOUT A SCALE

One of the first things you'll need to do when you start Step One is to push your scale to the back of a deep closet and forget about it for eight weeks. During that time, your body will be adjusting to an entirely new way of losing weight. You will see tremendous progress and weight loss as you finish Step One and, later, Step Two. But if you stick to the traditional means of measuring weight loss on a day-to-day basis, you will suffer unnecessary frustrations.

Over their lifetime, many people with Metabolism B have gained, lost, and regained hundreds of pounds, following diets written for people with Metabolism A. The scale has always been the traditional gadget to track progress on a typical weight-loss diet that emphasizes limiting and burning calories. So dieters dutifully weigh themselves every day, coming away with a number that can lift them high or plunge them into despair.

I sometimes think of scales as "instruments of torture." Some of my patients admit to weighing themselves as often as three times a day. They remove earrings, watches, wallets, keys, and shoes before stepping on the scale. About a third close their eyes during their weigh-in, and some face backward to avoid seeing the number. Whether or not they are compulsive weighers or despise seeing their weight, the number on the scale is a source of anxiety.

For those with Metabolism B, stepping on a scale every day is not an accurate measure of progress. Most of their excess weight comes in the form of abdominal fat and is a result of the body's improper handling of carbohydrate caused by a hormonal imbalance. Your weight loss will have dips and pauses that will frustrate you if you rely on a day-to-day scale reading to measure your progress.

People assume when they are "on a diet" that their weight will very systematically decrease. In reality, if they plot their daily weight loss, one of three patterns will emerge. Each pattern, shown below, shows a very different outcome and can tell you a lot about your metabolism and health.

The Staircase (Metabolism A)

This type of *plateau weight loss* is the norm and typifies weight loss for people with Metabolism A who follow traditional calorie-controlled diets. The graph resembles a set of stairs, with a few days of weight loss followed by a few days without loss. While on the plateau, weight loss temporarily slows or stops for days or even a week. Plateaus often discourage dieters, so they abandon their programs.

In actuality, a plateau is quite a healthy weight-loss pattern. It occurs when the brain, working like a sensor, detects weight loss and slows the loss until it can assess all of your bodily functions. Once it ascertains that you are healthy, it will allow further weight loss until the next check. In this way, the brain can slow starvation or allow healthy weight loss.

The Ski Slope

This pattern represents *uncontrolled weight loss*. Starting weight is the top of the slope, and it continues to decline, uninterrupted. Although this is the type of weight loss most people seek, they don't realize that unchecked weight loss is *not* normal. It often indicates a medical concern such as hyperthyroidism, uncontrolled diabetes, cancer, or gastrointestinal conditions, and it is a red flag for health-care providers.

Solo Measurements

If you are taking measurements for yourself, fasten the end of the tape measure to your skin with a piece of tape to hold it in place, as another set of hands would.

ᘯᘓ The Descending Curlicue (Metabolism B)

The weight loss of people with Metabolism B is *hormonal*. You do not experience weight loss in neat steps but, rather, in a very erratic pattern that occasionally shows you gaining weight even as you average a solid weight loss. Because of this erratic pattern, I recommend weighing and measuring yourself only after your eight weeks on Step One and once a month thereafter. Note your starting weight, and, at the end of the eight weeks or month, when you get back on the scale, you will be thrilled with your progress. In this way, you'll be spared the frustrating ups, downs, and curlicues that occur in between. At the end of this chapter, we have provided a chart where you can check your weight loss at the end of eight weeks with how many pounds we expect you to lose, based on your sex, height, and weight.

TRUST YOUR MEASURING TAPE

In lieu of scale weighing, measure progress in inches with a fabric tape measure (buy one at a local fabric or discount store). The inches of fat that you lose around your belly and other areas of your body will impress you even more than the number on the scale will.

Measure yourself at the start of the program and monthly thereafter. Most people get measured by a spouse, a partner, a friend, an older child, or an assistant at a gym. The person who does your initial body measurements should be the same person who performs the measurements each time, as everyone has his or her own touch with a measuring tape.

Keep a month-to-month log of the following measurements.

AREAS TO MEASURE	MONTH 1 (DATE)	MONTH 2 (DATE)	MONTH 3 (DATE)_
Neck			
Chest (fullest area)			
Women (bra line)			
Waistline			
Hips (fullest area)			
Right thigh			
Left thigh			
Right calf (midway between knee and ankle)			
Left calf			
Right ankle			
Left ankle			
Right upper arm (midway between elbow and shoulder)			
Left upper arm			
Right wrist			

WHAT'S WRONG WITH WEIGHT CHARTS AND BMIS?

Americans love a good chart, and we take particular pleasure (or displeasure) in finding ourselves on the spectrum and comparing ourselves to others. But "ideal body weight" charts are extremely limited and sometimes deceptive in what they tell you. I never use them in my practice because they make no distinction between fat weight and muscle weight. Some people who rank heavier on the scale or weight chart are actually less fat and much healthier than their nonexercising but physically lighter counterparts.

Take a minute and compare the statistics of two men. If you look only at their age, height, weight, and frame, you might conclude that Ray is in better shape.

	JOSEPH	RAY
Age	52	52
Height	5'9"	5'9"
Frame	Medium	Medium
Weight	178 pounds	170 pounds
THE YIKES ZONE		
Waist	34	37
LDL	97	128
Blood pressure	120/72	142/92
Exercise*	5 times/week	None

* More than 30 minutes/day

What *Is* Your Ideal Weight?

Not a day passes in my weight-loss practice without someone asking, "What is my ideal weight?" Your ideal weight is the weight at which you:

1. Are healthy

2. Have lab work in the normal range, with as little medication as possible

3. Like the way you look and feel

When you've met your ideal weight, you are ready for Step Three, the maintenance phase of the Metabolism Miracle.

If You Insist . . .

If you insist on weighing yourself daily, use this suggestion. For people with Metabolism B, day-to-day weigh-ins will make no sense because the weight loss follows no pat formula. Average your weekly weights, and compare one week's average to the next week; you'll have a better idea of how you are doing.

Look at the following example of a Metabolism B dieter's daily weight fluctuations:

WEEK 1 (POUNDS)	WEEK 2 (POUNDS)
Monday: 202	Monday: 200
Tuesday: 202.5	Tuesday: 199
Wednesday: 200.5	Wednesday: 198
Thursday: 199.5	Thursday: 197.5
Friday: 201	Friday: 198.5
Saturday: 199.5	Saturday: 197.5
Sunday: 199	Sunday: 197.5

The day-to-day loss is confusing. Now look at the difference between the person's two weeks' averages:

WEEK 1 (POUNDS)	WEEK 2 (POUNDS)
200.5	198

When this dieter compares his average weight from one week against his average weight the next, the loss is clear: 2.5 pounds.

Look a little deeper, at their respective waist measurements, blood work, and activity levels, and you come to a very different conclusion: Joseph is much healthier and thinner. Weight charts that offer only a piece of the picture don't tell the whole story.

Another chart system, the BMI (body mass index), promoted as a more accurate assessment of weight and fat than scale weight, divides your current weight by your height. But the concept has problems: It does not distinguish between gender, age, or physical activity level. Instead, it tosses everyone into the same pot, comparing men and women, young and old, active and inactive.

The BMI divides results into categories, with the normal range falling between 20 and 25, overweight considered falling between 25 and 30, and obesity starting at 30 and up. Using the BMI's simple comparison of weight to height, you would use the same chart to find the BMI of a young male athlete and an elderly woman. That means that you might compare a five-foot-nine, eighteen-year-old male wrestler to a five-foot-nine, seventy-five-year-old, extremely sedentary grandmother.

With your Metabolism B, place your trust in a *monthly* assessment with the measuring tape and scale. If you have uncontrolled type 2 diabetes or elevated blood sugar, cholesterol, or triglycerides, you'll also measure your

Starting Too High

Many people begin this program with excess glucose or lipids (fats) in their blood-stream. Those levels can sometimes alter the speed of the response that you see when you start the Miracle. If you are beginning the Metabolism Miracle with any of the following conditions, please read on.

Uncontrolled type 2 diabetes or elevated blood sugar: People with diabetes or prediabetes are usually familiar with the lab test called hemoglobin A1C (HbA1C). This blood analysis is taken quarterly and can estimate your average blood glucose for twenty-four hours per day, three months previous to the blood draw. If you begin the Miracle with HbA1C greater than 6.0, your body will consume excess blood glucose in the beginning stages of this program. Depending on how high your HbA1C is at the start of the program, it will take a little longer for your body to slip into the fat-burning mode. If you do not have diabetes or you have excellent control of your diabetes (HbA1C less than 6.0), there will be no excess sugar to consume, and fat burning will begin immediately after day three of Step One.

High cholesterol or high triglycerides: If you start the Metabolism Miracle with elevations in LDL cholesterol or triglycerides, your body will consume this excess fat in the first few days of Step One. Once your body has finished burning those blood lipids, it can turn to your fat cells so that you can lose inches around your midline and other parts of your body.

If your lipids are in the normal range, fat burning will begin immediately after day three of Step One.

progress with your lab numbers. You'll be looking for these six results as you progress with the Miracle.

1. *Loss of inches*

2. *Loss of weight*

3. *Increase in energy and quality of life*

4. *Decrease in blood sugar (if previously elevated)*

5. *Decrease in blood lipids (if previously elevated)*

6. *Decrease in blood pressure (if previously elevated)*

REAL READER SUCCESS STORY
Danielle Cavalli

Since 2005, Danielle has lost seventeen pounds.

Favorite MM Recipes: Eggplant Rollatini (page 289), Zucchini Muffins (page 314)

In high school, Danielle was a varsity track athlete. Standing at five foot ten, she was always very lean and long due to all the training she did for track. As her freshman year at the University of Maryland progressed, she noticed a lot of fluctuation in her weight, even though worked out regularly and watched what she ate. "I would gain five pounds in a weekend, and then lose two the next day. That cycle continued for months," she says. By her sophomore year, she was working out up to three hours a day and eating fewer than 1,000 calories in an attempt to stop her weight gain: "My once-lean frame at 155 healthy pounds was now creeping close to the 180 mark on the scale, and I was devastated and spiraling down the path to an eating disorder."

It wasn't until she was diagnosed with polycystic ovarian syndrome (PCOS) in 2005 that she finally got closer to a solution. "I was introduced to Diane by my endocrinologist," Danielle says. "From the day I met Diane, not only did I have answers to my weight and health issues but I had solutions, and my life, my health, and my body changed!"

For Danielle, the most challenging part of the program has been timing her meals. "My biggest hurdle is fitting my meals into my workday because I'm on the go all the time. I have an alarm on my cell phone that goes off every four and a half hours to remind me to eat," she says. Danielle keeps snacks on hands for when she doesn't have time for a full meal. "I always carry some peanuts, cheese sticks, or pita chips with me," she says.

Her father also started eating the Metabolism Miracle way, so she loves to have dinner at her parents' house: "My mom is a fantastic cook, and she's adapted for us." Danielle's mom makes a lot of fish and substitutes spaghetti squash for traditional wheat pasta—moves that, along with the rest of the plan, have helped her dad drop twenty-five pounds, lower his cholesterol, and fight off the onset of diabetes. "I don't miss pasta, which is funny since I'm really Italian," Danielle says. When she is in the mood for some authentic Italian food, her go-to dishes are Eggplant Rollatini (page 289) and especially Easy Pizza (page 227). "I make that a lot when I'm in a pinch," she says.

Even though she has just about met her goal weight, Danielle feels more comfortable living on Step Two of the plan. During the holidays, she tends to jump onto Step Three, but she usually goes back to Step One for eight weeks shortly after, resetting the process and bringing her back up to Step Two. "I'm very happy with where I'm at," she says. "I feel good. I'm a lot leaner now, so I can allow myself to go off the plan for a little while and get back on."

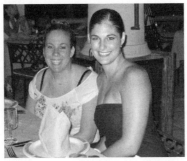
Before

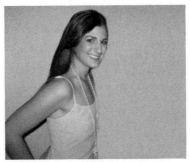
After

Most important, Danielle has learned how to manage her weight and her PCOS symptoms in healthy ways: "Knowing I have the power to regulate this on my own and take charge of it instead of letting it take charge of me is fantastic."

Danielle's Advice

"I went through hell and back trying to figure out what was wrong with me. I was in the gym four to five hours a day, not eating, and allowing myself to completely deteriorate. For girls in the same situation, I say, 'Go see Diane. She will fix it.' Knowing there are great solutions makes this something I'm very open about."

EXCEPTIONAL FARE:
VEGETARIANS, DINING OUT,
HEALTHY SHOPPING LIST
FOR STEP ONE

Everyone has preferences when it comes to food. I see a lot of "meat and potatoes" folks in my practice, but I also see a good number of vegetarians and people who eat out more often than not. These patients usually express concern that they won't be able to follow the Metabolism Miracle. Nothing could be further from the truth.

VEGETARIAN FARE

The different varieties of vegetarianism all come with their own challenges. Ovo-lacto (eggs- and dairy-eating) vegetarians eat fruits, vegetables, grains, soy products, legumes, eggs, and dairy products, but they don't eat animal flesh, such as meat, fish, and poultry. On the other end of the spectrum, vegans exclude all animal products, including dairy and even honey. Some people consider themselves vegetarians when they avoid eating red meat. I call that simply the preference to avoid red meat.

Most vegetarian diets tend to be high in carbohydrates because vegetarians often build their base from fruit, starchy vegetables such as corn and potatoes, legumes such as lentils and chickpeas, and grains such as whole-grain rice, breads, and crackers. All of these foods are carbohydrates.

Vegetarians who were born with Metabolism A can lose weight on a low-calorie lifestyle that excludes such foods as fatty meats, cheeses, butter, and other dairy. Their body follows the traditional weight-loss formula that says if you take in fewer calories than you burn, you will lose weight.

But that's not true for vegetarians who were born with Metabolism B. They are often perplexed by the fact that although they have purposely modified their lifestyle to avoid high-fat meats (and dairy, in the case of vegans), often, in an effort to lose weight and decrease cholesterol, they find the exact opposite occurring. They have unwittingly replaced many proteins and fats with carbohydrates, and of course Metabolism B wreaks havoc when carbohydrates come into the body in large quantities and in an unscheduled time pattern.

For vegetarians who eat eggs and dairy, the solution lies in balancing the diet with high-value vegetarian proteins rather than depending solely upon carbohydrate. They can easily follow all the basic rules of every step of the Metabolism Miracle, enjoy their meals, and reap excellent results, losing weight and optimizing their health.

Vegans need slightly more planning to follow the Metabolism Miracle program. Because they rely completely on nonanimal and often high-carbohydrate sources of protein, and because Step One is an extremely low-carb phase, I recommend their diminishing the time spent on Step One to four weeks. During Step One, protein needs can be met with soy milk, tofu, soy products, nut butters, and nuts while the pancreas and liver rest. For a vegan, it's prudent to spend the rest of the weight-loss mode, for at least eight weeks, in Step Two, which will include minimal amounts of whole grains, legumes, and fruits. Stay in Step Two until you reach your desired weight.

Step Two is more reasonable for vegans because it introduces whole grains, such as whole wheat bread and brown rice, and legumes to the mix. If you are uncertain of how to adapt veganism to Steps One and Two of the Miracle, you might want to make a visit to a registered dietitian who can help you establish a plan week by week.

Sample Menus

Step One Ovo-Lacto Vegetarian Sample Menu

5:30 a.m.—Wake up

6:00 a.m.—Breakfast
Omelet with egg whites, light shredded Cheddar, peppers, onions, and tomatoes
1 slice low-carb bread (5 g net carb or less) (5 × 5 carb)
Whipped butter

Stephen: New to Vegetarianism . . . and Gaining Weight?

Stephen, a thirty-six-year-old computer programmer, had recently decided to become a vegetarian. A self-described environmentalist, he called the office to make an appointment, telling the receptionist that he did not eat "anything with a face."

Stephen was perplexed by a recent weight gain that occurred when he eliminated high-calorie protein products from his diet. He brought a detailed one-week food diary to our initial session, outlining meals with whole-grain breads and pastas, brown rice, legumes, fruit, juices, eggs, and cheese, milk, and other dairy products.

He asked me to configure his caloric intake, as he felt that what he was eating did not add up to his weight change. To maintain a healthful weight at his height, Stephen's calorie requirement was approximately 2,100 calories per day. Yet his food diary reported that he was eating about 1,400 calories a day. He should have been losing weight on this calorie amount, and yet, over the past six months, he had gained six pounds.

Stephen's new weight gain showed up right around his midline. He found himself winded when he walked up just two flights of stairs and was too tired to go out with friends on the weekend. His youngest sister was recently diagnosed with PCOS (polycystic ovarian syndrome), and his father, who had had type 2 diabetes, died of a heart attack in his early sixties. Lab work from the previous year showed that Stephen's glucose was 99 (normal is 65–99 mg/dL [3.6 mmol/L–5.5 mmol/L]). His lipids were within normal range, except for his LDL cholesterol at 117 (normal is less than 100).

9:00 a.m.—Midmorning snack

Part-skim string cheese and a handful of almonds

12:00 noon—Lunch

Meatless burger (no carbs) with Swiss cheese, shredded lettuce, sliced tomato, and onion, in a low-carb tortilla (5 g net carb or less) (5 × 5 carb)

Sugar-free ice pop

4:00 p.m.—Afternoon snack

Cottage cheese cup with tomato wedge

Handful of pumpkin seed kernels

I suspected that his labs had changed over the past twelve months and asked him to get new lab work for our first session. His glucose had risen to 102; triglycerides were 134; and his total cholesterol, LDL, and blood pressure had all increased. All the signs added up.

Stephen had Metabolism B, and it had begun to wreak havoc on his new *higher*-carbohydrate diet. His vegetarian diet choices, while lower in calories and fat, were much higher in total carbohydrate. Grains, legumes, fruits, and many milk products are mainly carbohydrates. His Metabolism B was overprocessing these foods and depositing fat around his middle and in his blood.

When Stephen looked at the list of foods he could eat during Step One, he didn't think he could make it through the eight weeks as a vegetarian because the list emphasized meat, fish, and poultry but nixed carbohydrate, the mainstay of his vegetarian menu. He was relieved to see that his protein needs could be met with eggs or egg whites, low-fat carb-controlled milk, low-fat cheese, soy products, tofu, nut butters, and protein drinks. He was also relieved that he could eat liberal amounts of many vegetables.

Within the first eight weeks, Stephen had lost the weight. By the time he finished Step Two, his lab work entered the normal zone. He had been able to easily maintain his eggs-and-dairy vegetarian lifestyle throughout all three steps of the Miracle. He lives on his maintenance plan and looks and feels great.

6:30 p.m.—Dinner

Miracle Quiche (recipe on page 219)

Large garden salad with balsamic vinaigrette

"Gilded" Cinnamon Muffin (recipe on page 313) (5 × 5 carb)

11:00 p.m.—Bedtime snack

Cinnamon Ricotta Pudding (recipe on page 315)

Step Two Ovo-Lacto Vegetarian Sample Menu

5:30 a.m.—Wake up

6:00 a.m.—Breakfast

Egg white omelet with light shredded cheese and veggies

1 light multigrain English muffin (11–20 g net carb serving) with
whipped butter

9:00 a.m.—Midmorning snack

Sweet Nut Treat (recipe on page 238) (11–20 grams net carb serving)

Flavored yogurt (11–20 g net carb serving)

12 noon—Lunch

Grilled cheese sandwich made with 2 slices of thin-sliced whole-grain
bread (11–20 g net carb serving), sliced cheese, whipped butter, and
tomato slices

Sugar-free gelatin cup with whipped topping

4:00 p.m.—Afternoon snack

1 cup cantaloupe (11–20 g net carb serving)

7:00 p.m.—Dinner

3 Eggplant Rollatini (recipe on page 289) with soy meatballs (11–20 g
net carb serving) and grated Parmesan cheese

Large garden salad with balsamic vinaigrette

Chocolate Ricotta Pudding (recipe on page 315)

10:00 p.m.—Bedtime snack

Zucchini Muffin (recipe on page 314) (5 × 5 carb)

1 cup fat-free milk (11–20 grams net carb)

Step One Vegan Sample Menu

6:00 a.m.—Wake up

7:00 a.m.—Breakfast

8 ounces natural soy milk

1 low-carb tortilla (5 g net carb or less) (5 × 5 carb) with natural peanut butter

10:00 a.m.—Midmorning snack

Soy cheese

Almonds

12:00 noon—Lunch

Tofu burger (containing no carb grams), topped with melted soy cheese, lettuce, tomato, and onion slices, on 1 slice low-carb bread (5 g net carb or less) (5 × 5 carb)

Celery sticks with natural almond butter

3:00 p.m.—Afternoon Snack

Crumbled tofu with roasted vegetables

Handful of sunflower kernels

5:00 p.m.—Dinner

Spaghetti squash with $\frac{1}{2}$ cup crushed-tomato marinara with Italian herbs and ground tofu browned in olive oil

1 slice low-carb "garlic bread" with olive oil and garlic (5 × 5 carb)

Large garden salad with balsamic vinaigrette

9:30 p.m.—Bedtime Snack

1 slice low-carb bread (5 × 5 carb) with natural peanut butter

1 cup soy milk

Step Two Vegan Sample Menu

7:00 a.m.—Wake up

7:30 a.m.—Breakfast

$\frac{1}{2}$ cup oatmeal (11–20 g net carb serving) with 1 cup soy milk, a sprinkle of cinnamon, and sliced almonds

1 piece low-carb toast (5 × 5 carb) with natural peanut butter

11:00 a.m.—Midmorning snack

1 apple (11–20 g net carb serving)
Handful of walnuts

2:00 p.m.—Lunch

Large salad containing crumbled tofu, sunflower seed kernels, veggie
"chicken" nuggets (5 g net carb or less) (5 × 5 carb), and $\frac{1}{2}$ cup
chickpeas (11–20 g net carb serving)
Olive oil and vinegar dressing

5:00 p.m.—Afternoon snack

Celery sticks with almond butter
1 fresh peach (11–20 g net carb)

8:00 p.m.—Dinner

Sliced Tofurkey (vegetarian tofu-based "turkey")
$\frac{1}{2}$ sweet potato (11–20 g net carb)
Large portion of steamed broccoli with olive oil and garlic
Salad with pumpkin seed kernels and vinaigrette

11:30 p.m.—Bedtime Snack

$\frac{1}{2}$ cup cereal (9 g net carb) with 1 cup unsweetened soy milk and
4 strawberries (9 g net carb) (total carb serving for the entire snack
should be between 11–20 g)

EATING IN RESTAURANTS

Many of my patients travel for their work or simply enjoy dining out
frequently. Using the same thoughtful choices that you put into home
meals, the Metabolism Miracle program will work well in any restaurant. Fine dining, take-out, and even fast-food choices are easy on all
three of the steps.

Step One: Be a bit of a purist during Step One. Order easy, single-entity
low-carb entrées such as chicken, veal, pork, or lean steak, rather than a
combination food or a choice with which you are unfamiliar. Avoid breadings and unknown sauces.

Because you don't have to count calories, portion sizes of protein choices
are not an issue. You can also indulge at the salad bar, enjoying double portions of grilled veggies, lettuce, peppers, and shredded cheese, eggs, olives,

sunflower seed kernels, and broccoli. Just stay away from higher-carb choices such as chickpeas, croutons, beets, kidney beans, fruit salad, pasta salad, and potato salad.

Steps Two and Three: It is even easier to eat out once you graduate to Steps Two and Three. You will be able to include breadings, sauces, and hidden cornstarch, counting them as single-carb servings. Just about any food can be worked into your recommended carb range when you are following the maintenance phase of the Miracle.

12 Tips for Eating Out, MM Style

1. **Check your watch.** Consider the number of hours between your last meal or snack and when your food will arrive at your table. If it will be close to or over the five-hour mark, remember to eat an appropriate snack to "dam" the liver from releasing excess sugar before you even get the chance to order.

2. **Have it your way.** Don't be timid about making reasonable requests, such as dressing on the side, an extra order of broccoli to replace the potato, or chicken breast without barbecue sauce. Keep in mind that many people have dietary considerations, and restaurants often fill special requests.

3. **Skip the bread.** Request that no bread or chip basket be brought to the table, or move the basket out of sight so it stays off your mind.

4. **Order simply.** Select unbreaded meat, fish, or poultry with vegetables and salad. Skip sauces, breadings, and gravies.

5. **Make salad considerations.** Avoid carrots and croutons in premade salads, as they contain unnecessary carbs.

6. **Replace starch with extra veggies.** Replace potato, rice, or pasta with an extra order of healthy vegetables.

7. **Find the carb-friendly menu section.** Many restaurants accommodate dieters, with low-carb sections on their menus.

8. **Check nutrient facts.** More and more restaurants now include nutrition facts on their menus (and some are even required by local health

regulations to do so). Use the formula to compare the carb and fiber grams with your carb needs (see "Net Carb Formula," page 55).

9. **Opt for meal salads.** A large salad with protein makes a great low-carb entrée. Choose chef's salad, antipasto, or chicken Caesar without croutons.

10. **Request a sandwich sans bread.** Ask for the "insides" of your favorite sandwich on top of a bed of salad greens with dressing on the side. Ask the waiter to hold the bread.

11. **Enjoy a burger with the fixings.** Enjoy the beef, cheese, lettuce, tomato, onion, and pickle without a bun.

12. **Have breakfast for lunch.** Have a western omelet (egg whites or egg substitute preferred) with cheese, vegetables, and Canadian bacon.

Chinese Food

Chinese food can be full of great vegetables and fresh ingredients, but rice and noodles make most Chinese dishes high in carbohydrate. During Step One, skip the rice, noodles, fried noodles, wontons, breadings, and most of the sauces, which often contain hidden carbohydrate in the form of cornstarch.

Think about hidden carbs when you make an order. Chicken and broccoli without the rice seems like a perfect choice to order for Step One, but the sauce often contains cornstarch. It's a fine choice for Steps Two and Three, when you count the sauce as a single carb serving. Order Chinese food with no sugar or starch when possible.

Chinese Food to Avoid

Rice (white rice, fried rice, steamed rice, rice balls)

Noodles (pasta, wontons, wrappers)

Sweet sauces (duck/plum sauce, sweet-and-sour sauce, oyster sauce, hoisin sauce)

The crispy covering of egg rolls

Breaded or coated meats (General Tso's chicken, for example)

Deep-fried items

Chinese Food to Enjoy

Soups (egg drop soup, chicken broth with scallions, hot-and-sour soup)

The inside of egg rolls (don't eat the wrappers)

Steamed foods without sauces: Order egg drop or chicken broth on the side, and use the soup as the sauce for a steamed dish.

Stir-fried dishes (without sugar or starch)

Mu shu (without the wrappers)

Egg foo yong (without gravy)

Mongolian barbecue (often present at Chinese buffets). Choose your own meats and veggies and request no sauce.

Italian Food

Mention Italian food and many people envision pasta, pizza, and crusty white bread. But real Italians don't load on the carbs as most Americans think. I remember my parents searching for a slice of pizza in Rome. What they found had a paper-thin crust, light tomato sauce, and very little cheese, nothing like the greasy concoction we call pizza in the USA.

Italian Food to Avoid

A tray of lasagna with a loaf of garlic bread can spell disaster for someone with Metabolism B. Instead, eat like true Italians, ordering fish or meat with pasta on the side in a small portion. Ask for pasta to be prepared al dente, which lowers its carbohydrate impact.

Italian Food to Enjoy

Antipasti: A typical antipasti platter (the term means "before the meal") contains an assortment of meats, cheeses, marinated veggies, and olives, all acceptable on any step of the Miracle. Other good appetizers include grilled, roasted, or marinated veggies; steamed clams or mussels; fresh mozzarella with tomatoes and basil; and shrimp sautéed in garlic and wine.

Soups (chicken broth with spinach, simple vegetable soup, Italian wedding soup without pasta, or Italian egg drop soup)

Salads: Most contain dark greens, olive oil, and crushed garlic. Feel free to add cheese and tomatoes, but skip the croutons.

Seafood (usually great choices, as are chicken and veal entrées with sauce on the side for flavor)

Pizza: If you crave pizza during Step One, satisfy that urge by enjoying the topping—cheese, onions, peppers, spinach, broccoli—and leaving the crust behind.

Mexican Food

By nature, Mexican food is steeped in carb, with its rice, beans, corn, tortillas, tacos, burritos, enchiladas, and tamales. But there are plenty of metabolism B–friendly choices to make in any Mexican restaurant. The trick is to count your carb servings and think about what's inside all of those tacos, tortillas, and other wraps.

Mexican Food to Avoid

Hold the rice, hold the tortilla chips. Remember to request "no rice" and shun the basket of tortilla chips. During Step Three, about twelve tortilla chips, $1/2$ cup of beans, or $1/3$ cup of rice = 1 carb serving.

Wraps, tortillas, and more. Most carbs in Mexican food come from tortilla shells, wraps, rice, and beans. Peek inside burritos, chimichangas, enchiladas, tacos, tortillas, and the like to see if what's inside will work for you: seasoned taco meat, shredded cheese, lettuce, tomato, salsa, and sour cream are all fine, even during Step One.

One carb serving of 11–20 grams equals:

12 tortilla chips

$1/3$ cup rice

2 hard taco shells

1 soft taco shell

Mexican Food to Enjoy

Pass the guacamole and cucumber chips. Avocado is a heart-healthy fat and is fine during all steps of the Miracle. Use cucumber slices for dipping, or use a spoon.

"Ensalada, por favor." A salad is a great appetizer choice. Skip the hard tortilla shell of the tostada salad . . . everything inside is great.

Grilled proteins and vegetables: Grilled seafood with a light salsa, carne asada (grilled steak with Mexican spices), and chicken dishes with grilled vegetables and salsas make very friendly fare for anyone with Metabolism B.

Fajitas: Even people on Step One can enjoy all of the fajita accompaniments (shrimp, steak, chicken, guacamole, cheese, salsa, sour cream, tomato, lettuce, and onion), but skip the soft tortilla shells. During Step Three, each fajita shell = 1 carb serving.

Machaca. This common breakfast of eggs, beef, and vegetables works for Steps One, Two, and Three.

Fast Food

Fast food is always a dubious choice for anyone on a diet. But you can make decent choices when you're following the Metabolism Miracle and you find yourself at a fast-food restaurant.

Fast Food to Avoid

Skip breaded chicken and fish. Although both are lean proteins, chicken and fish when coated with a breading and then deep-fried take on extra carbs and fat.

Skip fries, tots, onion rings, and shakes. They have astronomical amounts of carb, fat, and calories.

Fast Food to Enjoy

Grilled chicken: Along with cheese, lettuce, and tomato, grilled chicken makes a great meal.

Grilled burgers: Top a grilled burger with cheese and plenty of lettuce, tomato, onions, and pickles. Skip the bun.

Salads: Many fast-food restaurants now offer salads that feature protein, such as chicken or steak, cheese and eggs. Opt for low-fat dressing or vinaigrette.

Shed the shell: The inside of tacos works well as a meal, but toss out the shell.

McMuffin without the muffin: Order breakfast egg sandwiches without the bread, or toss it out once you open the wrapper.

Go inside the sub: Skip the roll and turn the interior of a submarine sandwich— the ham, cheese, turkey, roast beef, lettuce, tomato, oil, and vinegar—into a great salad.

Everything in Moderation

Remember that Steps One and Two are meant to be fat-burning phases. If you consume greasy, high-fat food, your body will waste time burning the fat from the cheeseburger before it can get around to burning the fat from you. Limit fast foods, even low-carb choices, for the quickest weight loss.

AT-A-GLANCE SHOPPING LIST FOR STEP ONE

Asterisked items (*) represent 5 × 5 carbs—check the label to make sure they don't exceed 5 grams of net carbs.

Beverages: sugar-free flavored water, sugar-free iced tea mix, sugar-free soda sweetened with Splenda, sugar-free hot cocoa mix, club soda, flavored seltzer, coffee, tea

Green tea bags

Supplements: multivitamin, 500–600 mg calcium with vitamin D, 1,000–1,200 mg fish oil or flaxseed oil capsules, vitamin E (check dosage in multivitamin and add separate vitamin E capsule to total 400 IU)

Protein drinks* (should have *less than* 5 g net carb)

Peanut or nut butter: natural peanut butter or almond butter

Cheese: reduced-fat string cheese, part-skim string cheese, part-skim ricotta cheese, part-skim mozzarella cheese, 2% reduced-fat Cheddar cheese, 2% American cheese, Lorraine Swiss cheese, low-fat cheese wedges and spreadable cheese, grated Parmesan cheese, 1–2% cottage cheese, any low-fat cheese

Nuts and peanuts: almonds, pecans, walnuts, cashews, pistachios, peanuts

Butter or margarine: whipped butter, butter blends (combination of butter and oil), tub margarine with "liquid oil" and no hydrogenation

Cream cheese: whipped or reduced-fat cream cheese

Meats: lean cuts of meat such as sirloin, 85–93% ground beef, ground round, ground sirloin, flank steak, London broil, T-bone, porterhouse

Poultry: skinless chicken breast, turkey breast, turkey bacon, turkey sausage

Fish: any fish or shellfish

Pork: lean cuts such as tenderloin, center-cut loin chops, Canadian bacon, ham

Eggs: organic eggs, egg whites, egg substitutes such as Egg Beaters

Soy products: tofu, unsweetened soy milk, meat substitutes

Vegetables*: fresh or frozen artichokes, green beans, broccoli, cauliflower, spinach, lettuce, tomatoes, zucchini, summer squash, spaghetti squash, onions, peppers, mushrooms, bean sprouts, celery, cabbage, cucumber, eggplant, endive, chard, collards, kale, vegetable juice*, tomato juice*, asparagus, Brussels sprouts

Milk*: low-carb milk (5 g net carb or less)

Creamer: low-fat half-and-half or light cream

Sour cream: light or low fat

Salad dressing: olive oil and balsamic vinegar, low-fat* or light* salad dressing

Oils: olive, canola, peanut, safflower, sunflower, corn, vegetable

Cooking oil spray Mayonnaise: light or low-fat preferred

Bread: low-carb bread*, low-carb tortilla* (5 g net carb or less)

Yogurt: low-carb yogurt* (5 g net carb or less)

Jelly: sugar-free* (5 g net carb or less)

Syrup*: sugar-free* (5 g net carb or less)

Broth or bouillon

Lemon or lime juice

Condiments: low-carb* or sugar-free* ketchup, mustard, dill pickles

Splenda: packets and granulated

Sweets: sugar-free ice pops*, sugar-free gelatin, light* whipped cream, sugar-free* puddings* (5 g net carb or less)

REAL READER SUCCESS STORY
Nancie Bartie

Since September 2009, Nancy has lost thirty pounds.

Favorite MM Recipes: Pesto Cherry Tomatoes (page 242)

"Since starting MM, I've regained all my confidence," says Nancy Bartie, a kindergarten teacher in Minnesota. In 1978, Nancy was a Philadelphia Eagles cheerleader who, at five foot three, weighed 117 pounds. After her pregnancies and thirty years away from the football field, she was struggling to stay below 150 pounds. Although she was eating healthy and thought she was doing everything right, the number on the scale wouldn't budge.

In September 2009, she attended a thirty-year reunion with the Philadelphia Eagles cheerleaders. "As a size 6, I looked puffy," she recalls. However, she was already on the road to change. Just a few weeks prior, she had started the Metabolism Miracle.

"Once I started MM, all the weight came off quickly. Within twenty-four hours, I no longer had any carb cravings. Because I immediately had more energy and it was real food and all delicious, I felt satisfied," she says. "For years I thought I was eating healthy, but I didn't have the right tools. Fruit was my biggest downfall. I would even count the pretzels, thinking I was healthy, but it was too many carbs for me, I found out from the book."

As a kindergarten teacher, Nancy stayed engaged in the eating plan by keeping it fun: "I make it a game. My carbs are not my enemy. At each meal, once every five hours, I choose: Do I want what's behind door number one, two, or three? Do I want three-quarters cup of grapes, a slice of bread, or an ounce of dark chocolate?"

Now in Step Two, Nancy has lost thirty pounds. She says that she gets stopped often in the grocery story by people she hasn't seen in a while. They'll look at her; peer into her cart piled high with veggies, nuts, and low-fat string cheese; and ask her how they can do it, too.

She doesn't promote her eating plan only in the grocery store. In August 2010, she began hosting a local radio show, and she always gets a flood of calls and letters when she brings up the Metabolism Miracle.

Nancy spreads the word with good reason: The plan has reshaped not only her health and figure but also her husband and even her dog Jack. "My dog's energy levels have increased, and his coat is so shiny," she says, explaining that she mixes a little of her Metabolism Miracle food in with his regular dog food. Jack aside, she is amazed at the changes she has seen in herself. Her blood work has never looked better, she is full of energy, and she is now back down to her 1978 cheering weight: "I am shocked. At my age, I never thought it would happen. To be back in my cheerleader shape at fifty-two—who would've thought I could recapture my youth?"

A year after Nancy began the eating plan, she joined in another reunion with the Eagles cheerleaders. "Here I was with my MM

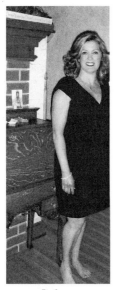

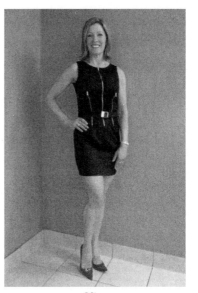

Before   After

healthy snack, and all the cheerleaders gathered round and said, 'That's how you do it? Tell us more,'" she says. Now some of them have started Metabolism Miracle, including one particular friend and former cheerleader. "This is her fourth week on Step One, and I check in with her every day," she says.

Nancy's new goal is to maintain her weight loss: "Three cheers if I fit into my wedding gown and maintain my desired weight as we celebrate our thirtieth wedding anniversary!"

Nancy's Advice

How to dine out: "Even at a restaurant, I'm able to pick and choose off the menu. I can order my protein and my vegetable, and then I bring six crackers in a plastic bag, knowing that those meet the Metabolism Miracle goal."

How to travel: "When I travel with a suitcase, I take my favorite MM food: the crackers that I know will meet the carb requirements for Step Two. I count out six, and if I'm going to be gone for seven days, I take seven plastic bags of these crackers. From the moment I step off the airplane, I'm ready to run and have fun because I bring the food with me."

PART THREE

Exploring Health and Life Issues

12

THE DIABETES CONNECTION

A family history of blood sugar–related problems holds a strong link to Metabolism B. If you or a close relative has had or currently has any of the following conditions, place a "check" before the line. See "A Blood Sugar Primer" (page 188) for a description of each condition.

_____ Low blood sugar (hypoglycemia)

_____ Gestational diabetes (diabetes related to pregnancy)

_____ Prediabetes (borderline diabetes)

_____ Type 2 diabetes (adult-onset diabetes)

There is a very definite link between a personal or family history of blood sugar abnormalities and Metabolism B. If you have had or currently have hypoglycemia, prediabetes, gestational diabetes, or type 2 diabetes, the Metabolism Miracle program will work for you with success where other weight-loss programs have failed.

If you have no personal history of these blood sugar conditions but a close family member does, you may still have inherited the gene for Metabolism B. Don't wait for a diagnosis of medical problems to develop over time. Use the Metabolism Miracle program to help prevent them.

Remember that people with Metabolism B cannot lose weight and keep it off following diets written for "normal" metabolism (Metabolism A). *The Metabolism Miracle* will work for you because it was written for you!

If you or a close relative has type 2 diabetes, the Metabolism Miracle can help you to permanently lose weight, control blood sugar, and impede the progression of this condition.

A Blood Sugar Primer

The food you eat provides your body with fuel in the form of *blood sugar*, also known as *blood glucose*. Your body strives to keep its fuel at the right concentration, somewhere between the normal range of 65 and 140 milligrams per deciliter (mg/dL), or 3.6 and 7.8 mmol/L. If blood glucose ventures outside of the target range, the entire body, and especially the brain, is forced to run on the wrong strength fuel, and health can suffer as a consequence.

Low Blood Sugar (Hypoglycemia)

There are two types of hypoglycemia. The first type, which can happen in a person with Metabolism B, occurs about one and a half to three hours after a carb-containing meal, due to the body's overrelease of insulin. Low blood sugar causes the person to feel dizzy, light-headed, nauseated, shaky, irritable, panicky, and ravenously hungry for carbohydrate food. Within a few minutes of eating carbohydrate, the symptoms subside. People with hypoglycemia often carry food with them "in case of emergencies" and declare to their friends, "We *need* to eat, now!"

Sudden mood swings and irritability often cue their friends that they mean business. This type of hypoglycemia is considered a precursor to prediabetes and type 2 diabetes.

The other type of hypoglycemia is medication induced. It occurs when a person with diabetes who takes oral medication or insulin injections to lower blood sugar experiences blood sugar below the normal range. People on glucose-lowering medication for diabetes are strongly advised to carry glucose tablets or another source of fast-acting carbohydrate.

Gestational Diabetes (Diabetes Related to Pregnancy)

About 6 percent of pregnant women develop high blood glucose between weeks 24 and 28 of pregnancy. Diet changes, exercise, and, in some cases, insulin injections are used to keep the condition under control until delivery, when most glucose levels return to normal. Babies born to women with uncontrolled gestational diabetes often tip the scales at close to or over nine pounds. These women have a greater chance of a subsequent pregnancy with gestational diabetes and of developing type 2 diabetes in the future.

A Touch of Sugar (Prediabetes)

Think of prediabetes as a red-flag alert. Also known as *borderline diabetes* or "a touch of sugar," this gray area between perfectly normal blood sugar and a diagnosis of type 2 diabetes offers a chance to prevent or at least slow down the progression with appropriate diet and exercise.

If you have prediabetes, you are lucky to have this opportunity to positively impact your medical future. The Metabolism Miracle is the only weight-loss program for you.

Type 2 Diabetes (Adult-Onset Diabetes)

Type 2 diabetes, also known as *adult onset diabetes*, comes from a combination of factors: a fatigued pancreas that can no longer produce enough insulin (the hormone that helps to ferry glucose from the blood into the cells for energy) and an increased resistance to that insulin from the very cells that need it.

After years of overproducing insulin during the prediabetes stage, the pancreas tires and begins to produce less and less of the hormone. Fat cells continually increase in size, and their insulin receptors distort as a result, making them resistant to the body's own insulin. Pressure then increases on the pancreas to produce more insulin, and this vicious cycle permanently impairs the pancreas's ability to produce enough insulin.

If you are overweight, inactive, and under mental or physical stress, and one of your parents has type 2 diabetes, your chances of developing the disease are high. When untreated or treated incorrectly, diabetes can cause irreversible and ongoing harm, including heart disease, blindness, nerve damage, and kidney damage. The good news is that even with a genetic predisposition to type 2 diabetes, you can improve your chances of avoiding this irreversible condition by losing weight, increasing physical activity, and reducing the stress in your life. And if you already have type 2 diabetes, you can control the condition with proper diet, physical activity, blood glucose monitoring, and medicine when required.

METABOLISM B AND TYPE 2 DIABETES

If you have had Metabolism B without knowing it or you've mistakenly followed traditional weight-loss programs while having Metabolism B, you have unknowingly increased your chances of developing type 2 diabetes. That's hard news if you have been doing your best to lose weight and take care of your body.

The good news is that by following the *appropriate* dietary program, you can delay or even prevent the development of type 2 diabetes. And if you already have type 2 diabetes, you can use the Metabolism Miracle to diminish the impact it has on your health, by controlling your blood sugar and symptoms and minimizing your need for medications.

It's important to recognize the signs of type 2 diabetes, a chronic, irreversible disease that usually occurs in combination with elevated LDL

Guidelines for Treating Hypoglycemia Caused by Diabetes Medication

IF BLOOD SUGAR IS LESS THAN 50 MG/DL (2.8 MMOL/L), CHOOSE ONE:

6–8 glucose tabs or
1 cup (8 ounces) of juice or
2 cups of nonfat milk or
12 ounces (1 can) of regular soda

IF BLOOD SUGAR IS 50–70MG/DL (2.8 MMOL/L–3.9 MMOL/L), CHOOSE ONE:

3–4 glucose tabs or
½ cup (4 ounces) juice or
1 cup nonfat milk

After you treat the hypoglycemia, wait fifteen minutes, retest, and confirm that blood sugar is once again in the 80–120 mg/dL range (4.4–6.7 mmol/L). If it remains under 70 mg/dL (3.9 mmol/L), re-treat as above and test again in fifteen minutes. Be sure to inform your physician of your hypoglycemic reaction for a possible medication decrease.

cholesterol, triglycerides, hypertension, and weight issues. Some of the common warning signs of the disease include:

● Increased thirst

● Increased urination

● Increased hunger

● Blurry vision

Many people walk around with diabetes for years before they are medically diagnosed. Although diabetes occurs when fasting blood sugar exceeds 125 mg/dL (6.9 mmol/L), the warning signs rarely surface until blood sugar exceeds 200 mg/dL (11.1 mmol/dL). I work with an endocrinologist who automatically tacks five years onto the date of a person's diabetes diagnosis. He believes that it takes about five years from when blood sugar initially exceeds 125 mg/dL to when that person feels ill and seeks medical attention.

A diagnosis of type 2 diabetes is usually made when two fasting blood glucose readings are shown to be *more than* 126 mg/dL (7 mmol/L).

Type 2 diabetes carries the potential for a number of life-threatening health consequences down the road, including blindness, kidney failure, heart attack, stroke, amputation, and nerve disorders. To understand how years of high blood glucose causes so much damage, you must look inside the blood vessels.

Regardless of what they eat or drink, the blood sugar of people without glucose problems will never exceed 140 mg/dL (7.8 mmol/L). By contrast,

	NORMAL	PREDIABETES	TYPE 2 DIABETES
Fasting blood sugar (in mg/dL)	65–99	100–125	Greater than 126*
2 hours after eating (in mg/dL)	Less than 140	Greater than 140 but less than 200	Greater than 200

*Type 2 diabetes is most often diagnosed by fasting blood glucose.

people with prediabetes or diabetes frequently have blood glucose above 140. This supersaturated blood sugar paints the lining of every blood vessel with a syrupy coating.

The sticky, sugarcoated walls of blood vessels act like glue for excess LDL and triglycerides. Remember that people with untreated Metabolism B typically have elevated blood lipids. It's no wonder that a person with type 2 diabetes has a 50 percent greater chance of suffering a heart attack or stroke than does a nondiabetic person. The thicker the deposits of fat become, the narrower the diameter of the blood vessel. Eventually, the individual accumulates a significant blockage that can ultimately lead to a heart attack or stroke.

In addition, blood vessels should be flexible and bend like a well-cooked strand of spaghetti. The blood vessels of a person with uncontrolled diabetes will harden and may break or have jagged edges that catch circulating fats like a dam blocks a stream and cause inflammation that has been linked to heart disease.

It is this damage to the blood vessels and nerves that leads to each of the following health-threatening complications of diabetes.

Retinopathy: Tiny blood vessels in the retina of the eye harden and eventually break and hemorrhage and can lead to blindness.

Neuropathy: Nerve endings that have been exposed to high levels of sugar for a period of time can harden, decreasing the nerve's ability to transfer impulses. Such damage can lead to hypersensation, lack of sensation, digestive problems, irregular heartbeat, sexual dysfunction, and more.

Nephropathy: Year after year, elevated blood sugar hardens the small blood vessels of the kidney, causing them to snap. Broken blood vessels impede the kidney's ability to filter toxins from the blood. As filtering ability decreases, toxins and waste products build up in the blood and may lead to the need for renal dialysis.

Circulatory problems: Because your feet contain the vessels furthest from the heart, vessel damage from plaque and hardening impede circulation and deaden nerves. Antibiotics may not be able to reach an infection in the feet and legs. Serious circulatory problems can lead to amputations.

IT'S ALL ABOUT CONTROL

Complications from diabetes occur *only* when the disease goes uncontrolled. The Metabolism Miracle gives you the knowledge and skills to control the two main components of type 2 diabetes—insulin resistance and a burned-out pancreas.

People with Metabolism B are born with a genetic propensity to over-release insulin in response to a rise in blood sugar. Remember that insulin is the hormone responsible for ferrying blood glucose into the muscle and fat cells of the body. When an event or hormonal change in the life of someone with Metabolism B triggers the pancreas to manifest this hyper-insulin release, it eventually leads to weight gain. The more weight that people with Metabolism B gain, the higher their risk of developing insulin resistance.

As you gain weight, your fat cells get larger in size. When you lose weight, they decrease in size. Both fat and muscle cells have receptors for insulin to attach and open the cell for glucose. Insulin acts like a key, fitting the receptor keyholes. The insulin receptors of people with Metabolism A will remain constant in shape no matter how large their fat cells become. But when people with Metabolism B gain weight, the fat cells stretch, and their insulin receptors warp to the point that the key no longer fits the keyhole. When this happens, such people are now resistant to their own insulin.

First Things First

Before beginning any diet or exercise program, contact your physician. This is particularly important if you have diabetes and are taking oral medication or insulin to control blood sugar. The Metabolism Miracle will help you to lose weight and decrease blood sugar, blood pressure, and blood lipids, and those changes may warrant a change in your medication or dosage.

Keep your doctor abreast of weight losses of ten pounds or more, and always report symptoms that might indicate overmedication.

The cell sends a message to the brain that it is hungry and needs insulin to open its door and usher in the glucose. The brain keeps calling on the pancreas to release insulin. The pancreas obliges, but because the insulin keys can't fit properly into the keyhole receptors, the glucose rarely gets into the cell. The brain calls on the pancreas over and over again. Eventually the pancreas fatigues to the point of exhaustion, cells are underfed, sugar backs up in the bloodstream, and you have the beginning of type 2 diabetes.

STOP THE TRAIN

Think of type 2 diabetes as a runaway train. It is best to stop the train in its tracks as early as possible. When detected early, diabetes can be successfully treated with diet and exercise. Unfortunately, the traditional diet for diabetes will speed up the pancreas burnout and the stretching of the insulin receptors. The traditional American Diabetes Association diet recommends a meal plan that contains about 50 to 55 percent carbohydrate. As you know, 100 percent of carbohydrate converts to blood sugar and causes the pancreas to release insulin. The main nutrient in the traditional diet for diabetes is the one nutrient that the person with diabetes cannot handle effectively.

When the traditional diet fails to control blood sugar in type 2 diabetes, the next step is to take oral medications. Keep in mind that the traditional diet overworks the pancreas with its excessive amount of carbohydrate. The oral diabetes medications that can lower blood glucose are medications that force the pancreas to release even more insulin. The very medication prescribed to lower blood sugar is medication that will speed up the burnout of the pancreas. Once the pancreas is burned out, no amount of oral medication can squeeze more insulin from the pancreas. At this point, the only option is injecting insulin for the rest of the person's life.

There is a way to stop the train. If you have Metabolism B and follow the Metabolism Miracle program as a way of life, you will absolutely lose weight. Your pancreas will rest before it is irretrievably burned out. You will retrain your pancreas to react normally to blood glucose changes. As you lose weight, your insulin receptors will regain their original shape. You can prevent or greatly forestall the onset of type 2 diabetes. If you already have type 2 diabetes and you follow the Metabolism Miracle way of life, you can actually prevent complications or forestall the need for insulin injections, effectively stopping the runaway metabolic train in its tracks.

WILL EVERY PERSON WITH METABOLISM B DEVELOP TYPE 2 DIABETES?

For a long time, the medical community thought that type 2 diabetes, hypertension, and high cholesterol came as the direct result of overeating and lack of physical activity. We now know that the genetic predisposition for excess insulin release and insulin resistance starts this process for people with Metabolism B.

Everyone with Metabolism B has the *potential* to develop type 2 diabetes, but not everyone will. You cannot develop type 2 diabetes without the genetic predisposition for the disease—the same predisposition as Metabolism B. Think of diabetes as the last stop of the Metabolism B train. It appears that a combination of being born with the gene and environmental stressors moves the train through the stops of midline weight, to elevated blood pressure, to elevated lipids, to elevated blood sugar, and to type 2 diabetes. When a person who is born with Metabolism B is exposed to certain environmental triggers, his or her chances of developing type 2 diabetes will increase.

The greater the number of environmental factors that the person with Metabolism B is exposed to, the greater are his or her chances of developing diabetes.

When a person is diagnosed with type 2 diabetes, his or her midline weight is often at its highest point, coupled with physical activity at an all-time low. Stress may have recently increased or been occurring for an extended period of time. Add an illness as fleeting as a flu to the mix, and the chance of the symptoms progressing goes up even further.

THE DIABETES SETUP

This chart lists the combination of factors that conspire to trigger type 2 diabetes. If you have the gene for Metabolism B, any of the following environmental factors may usher you toward developing type 2 diabetes.

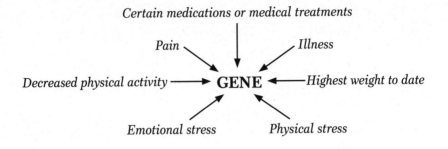

Given the conditions that may trigger diabetes, it makes wise sense for anyone with Metabolism B, and thus the chance of developing type 2 diabetes, to reduce weight with the appropriate diet, increase physical activity, learn to manage stress, and stay as healthy as possible.

The Metabolism Miracle helps you to beat the odds.

13

TRANSFORMATIONS: STORIES FROM THE FIELD

One of the truths about Metabolism B is that it affects so many different types of people in so many different walks of life. I've seen thousands of patients over the past twenty-five years, and since the development of this program, I've watched a lot of transformations take place as the Metabolism Miracle begins to work its magic. The following stories represent just a few of the many different people whom this program has helped usher from despair to empowerment.

MARGE, THE RETIRED NURSE

After years of procrastinating, sixty-nine-year-old Marge, a retired nurse, visited her orthopedic specialist to set up a date for knee replacement surgery. Marge had always been active, spending most of her working life on her feet. As a nurse at the community hospital, she stood for hours and felt the effects on her spine and joints. Still, she was surprised to learn that over the years her "good" knee had also deteriorated and she would require double knee replacements. To make matters worse, the doctor informed Marge that her blood sugar was borderline high and her blood pressure was slightly elevated.

Over the years, Marge had put on a few pounds and realized that the extra weight didn't help her joint pain. She attributed the weight gain to aging and the slower pace of her retired life. She hadn't worried about her weight until the surgeon told her to lose twenty pounds before he would operate.

Marge hobbled into my office, using a cane. She appeared older than her years and walked bent over with a limp, obviously in pain. She knew weight loss would help her properly rehabilitate after surgery but didn't know where to begin. She couldn't possibly exercise at this time and didn't see herself cooking elaborate meals or buying special foods.

Based on her diagnosis of prediabetes and hypertension, we decided the Metabolism Miracle matched her metabolism and would help her to lose weight quickly and permanently. It could also prevent her progression to type 2 diabetes, and the weight loss would help to lower her blood pressure.

I explained that meal preparation need not be cumbersome and that many foods required very little preparation, such as an egg white omelet with low-carb toast, a wrap with tuna, a protein shake and a handful of almonds, or cottage cheese and veggies or low-carb yogurt with a Miracle-recipe muffin. Marge would exercise using light hand weights and do muscle-toning activities in an armchair until she followed the prescribed physical therapy after surgery. She was pleased to learn that it wasn't about how many calories were burned; it was about energizing muscle tissue.

After Step One and eight weeks on Step Two, with a weight loss of twenty-two pounds, Marge had her double knee replacement and began physical therapy until she was navigating independently. The recovery had interrupted her normal diet, and so Marge returned to ten days of Step One, followed by Step Two, until she reached her desired weight. She is now cane free and pain free and remains diabetes free. She uses Step Three, the maintenance phase of the Miracle, with brief intervals of Steps One and Two, to give her system an occasional cleansing.

DAVE, THE HIGH SCHOOL ATHLETE

When Dave first came to my practice, he was a junior in high school. An honor student and member of both the baseball and football teams, Dave was generally upbeat and motivated, and, although quiet, he enjoyed hanging out with his many friends.

At five foot ten and 185 pounds, Dave lifted weights between sports seasons and always considered himself to be "tight and muscular." He reported eating everything and anything, including favorite foods such as bagels, pizza, chicken fingers, subs, Chinese food, burgers, and fries, always washed down with cola or iced tea.

After football season junior year, Dave noticed he felt much less energetic. His parents figured that his long days, school, homework, and friends caused the problem. Dave knew it was more than that. He had trouble waking up and felt wiped out after breakfast, after lunch, when he got home from school, and after dinner. It seemed as if he sank every time he ate a meal. He also, for the first time, had difficulty concentrating in class. He not only felt fatigued, his mind wandered. He couldn't pay attention to lessons and, even after studying, he had difficulty recalling the information for exams. He began to depend upon energy drinks in the evening to help him stay focused. When his third-quarter grades arrived, it was obvious something was wrong. His grades had dropped from the honor roll to include several Cs.

In the weight room, Dave also felt the drain. He had less energy to lift weights before baseball season and noticed that his belly had begun to protrude. One of his friends remarked that Dave was getting a gut. He felt more interested in watching sports from the couch than he did about going to the batting cages to get ready for the season.

Concerned about his slumping grades and his unusual choice of choosing video games and television over being with his friends or playing sports, his mother scheduled an appointment with Dave's doctor. After some prodding, Dave told his doctor that he was drained and down in the dumps, had no desire to do the things he used to enjoy, and was having difficulty in school. On the surface this sounded like mild depression, but after ruling out mononucleosis and Lyme disease, lab tests revealed surprises for the physician. This young, athletic male had a fasting glucose of 115 mg/dL (normal is 65–99 mg/dL or 3.6–5.5 mmol/L), total cholesterol of 212 (normal is less than 200), and LDL cholesterol of 118 (normal is less than 100).

Dave came to my office with a diagnosis of prediabetes and hyperlipidemia. He also had a teenager's skepticism. But he did recognize Metabolism B in himself as we discussed his symptoms of fatigue, anxiety, poor short-term memory, belly fat, and irritability. Mostly he wanted his old life back. He promised to "give it a shot" but, as he left my office, I wondered if he was being sincere.

Step One was a challenge to a young man who ate out with friends on a regular basis. He explained to buddies that he was on a boot camp–style program. They thought it was cool that Dave could use his diet and exercise to resculpt and rebuild his body. He never mentioned to them that the real reason for his lifestyle change was elevated cholesterol, high blood sugar, and a growing midline paunch. Dave chose from any menu that came his way; even fast-food menus had possibilities. At the local fast-food joint, he'd order two large grilled burgers "his way" with cheese, tomato slices, onions, pickles, and no bun. He even asked for extra lettuce in place of the bun and could pick up his huge creation with no problem! A sugar-free soda capped the meal. If he was still hungry, he'd also order a chicken Caesar side salad in place of his fries. He loved the freedom of liberal portions of lean protein, healthy fat, vegetables, and protein shakes.

Within a few weeks, Dave felt and looked better. His friends and, most important, his girlfriends told him he looked great. He could already see the difference in his ability to concentrate, and he felt like his old self.

Over the summer, Dave completed Step Two, reentering a world in which he enjoyed hanging out with friends and playing Frisbee on the beach. He began his senior year on Step Three, maintenance, and he says he has permanently adopted the Miracle not as a diet but as a way of life. He intends to live his life healthy and happy.

KAREN AND THE WEIGHT OF FAMILY BAGGAGE

Karen, who was referred to my practice by her psychiatrist, was overweight as a child and remembers "being on a diet" since she was about seven years old. She has clear memories of her mother calling her chubby and critiquing her food choices in front of friends and family. To this day, she feels the tension with her mother and can't shed the feeling of that embarrassed, chubby child when she visits her parents' home.

When Karen went away to college, she was able to take control of her weight. She juggled work, school, and a busy lifestyle. Without a car, she walked everywhere on campus. She was known for her upbeat, sunny, positive personality and felt on top of the world and in control of her weight and life.

After graduation, she became a third grade teacher and married her college sweetheart. On the outside, her world appeared perfect: a bright, healthy, happy, married woman embarking on life and career.

But something changed in December of her first year as a teacher. Karen felt decidedly different. She woke up exhausted, even after enough sleep. She stopped for a bagel on the way to work but needed coffee to give her some zip. She began to feel anxious on the way to work and sometimes felt her heart race and a cold sweat form on her face before entering the classroom.

Right before recess, she would begin to feel shaky and found herself watching the clock, hoping she could make it until the bell rang. As soon as the children filed out of the classroom, she hurriedly ate a candy bar from her purse. The behavior embarrassed her, but she couldn't seem to control it. The same feeling happened when she came home from school in the afternoon. She found herself in the kitchen, opening cabinet after cabinet, eating a little of this and a little of that. Next came the refrigerator, and Karen couldn't stop herself from consuming anything—peanut butter, cheese, cake, or leftovers. She knew that this was not normal, but she couldn't stop.

After her afternoon binges, disgusted with what she had done, Karen would need a nap, and she noticed that after dinner she had to lie down again because of how wiped out she felt. Her husband washed the dishes and cleaned up the kitchen while Karen dozed in front of the television. When he went to bed for the night, she would wake up and snack again.

One morning before her shower, Karen was shocked by her reflection in the bathroom mirror. How had she not noticed her belly, love handles, and back fat? Why hadn't anyone told her? But that was exactly what she despised about her childhood: being reminded of her weight gain. She realized at that moment that she had a problem and needed help.

Karen made an appointment with a psychiatrist and a medical doctor who ordered lab work before he began working with her. He found telltale signs: Her glucose was 104 (normal is 65–99 mg/dL or 3.6–5.5 mmol/L), and her triglycerides, LDL cholesterol, and HbA1C were all elevated. Karen was dealing with a physical problem along with her psychological problems. He referred her to my office to learn about her dietary needs based on her metabolism. Until her excess insulin and insulin resistance were treated and her metabolism stabilized, no amount of psychotherapy could help.

Karen was thrilled to understand the physical reasons for her eating behaviors and eagerly made the diet and exercise changes on the Miracle. Now her lab numbers are under control, and, working in tandem with her psychiatrist, Karen has reached her desired weight and come to terms with how her childhood has affected her body image and eating patterns. She and her husband hope to have a child soon, so we will next meet to tailor her program for pregnancy and lactation.

JIM, TYPE 2 DIABETES, AND A HOVERING WIFE

When Jim's wife, Barbara, called my office to make an appointment for her husband, she sounded anxious and reported that she was "at the end of her rope" with Jim, who had recently retired and now spent much of his time at home.

Jim, a salesman who traveled from city to city, was self-motivated and independent and had been very effective in his job. Now that they spent almost every waking hour together, Barbara worried about how her husband took care of himself, and she was concerned about their future. For the first time since Jim's diagnosis with type 2 diabetes ten years before, Barbara could witness his entire day, from wake-up to bedtime.

Barbara walked into the office first, with Jim walking behind. She filled in the initial assessment form while Jim read *Newsweek*. She pulled his medication list from her wallet and asked the receptionist to make a copy for his chart.

The couple's dynamic continued during the beginning of Jim's initial session. Barbara had a copy of her husband's daily blood sugar log. Although I tried to direct the questions to him, his wife finished his sentences and filled in the gaps of his diet history. About thirty minutes into our session, Barbara left for the restroom. While she was gone, I asked Jim if he would mind if we spoke about his diabetes care one-on-one. He didn't seem to care either way. Barbara waited in the reception room.

Without interruption or distraction, Jim and I worked very well together. It often helps to explain diabetes in a very concrete way, using the analogy of the body as a car and the problems that would occur if the car was forced to run on diesel instead of unleaded fuel. Similar to keeping up a car's maintenance, Jim needed to check his blood sugar at least twice a day, fill the tank with the appropriate fuel (carb allotment), run the car daily (exercise), and keep records of maintenance (log book/food log). My job was to teach him to take the best care of his health so that he would "run smoothly" for many years to come.

Jim's maintenance plan included checking his blood sugar twice a day, logging his results, and thinking of possible explanations for the readings (food, lack of exercise, forgotten medication, or stress). He would also walk for thirty minutes daily and begin Step One of the Miracle. Since Barbara was in charge of the household's shopping, menus, and meal preparation, we invited her back into the session.

Jim explained that he was going to take care of the monitoring, exercise, logging, and medication and that he would like Barbara's help as they got acclimated to Step One of the program. Barbara seemed both relieved and put out that she would not be totally involved in the management of Jim's diabetes.

Jim e-mailed me his blood sugar readings on a weekly basis, with notations for exercise and the reasons he felt readings were out of range. A weekly food log showed that he was on target with his diet program. Occasionally, Barbara would e-mail a few questions. She also made note that Jim was in control and feeling and looking much better.

When the couple returned in eight weeks for follow-up, Jim held the door open for Barbara, filled in his follow-up form, and handed me his records. While he had learned what he needed to do to maintain his health and well-being, Barbara had learned to support Jim in his self-management and attended his sessions as a "second set of ears."

As time passed, Jim's doctor adjusted his medication for diabetes, based on his much improved blood sugar. He now maintains excellent blood sugar while living on Step Three of the Metabolism Miracle. He does daily physical activity, takes much less medication, and enjoys a less stressful home life.

ANDREA, 25 YEARS OLD AND CONSIDERING GASTRIC BYPASS SURGERY

Three years ago, a young woman appeared at my office to fulfill her surgeon's requirement that she meet with a registered dietitian before she could be scheduled for gastric bypass surgery.

Andrea was visibly upset. She made very little eye contact and seemed ashamed to find herself in this position. As we talked, she told me of her years as a track star in high school and the track scholarship she received that enabled her to attend a top university. During her junior year, she suffered an orthopedic injury that required several surgeries and abruptly ended her days of training and competing. Over the past four years, she had gained ninety-five pounds.

At twenty-five years of age, Andrea was five foot six. In her running days, she competed at a weight of 150 pounds, but with her muscular body she'd appeared much thinner. She asked if she could face backward when I got her initial weight, as she couldn't bear to see the scale. Because she had lost much of her muscle tissue and tone, she appeared even heavier than her current 245 pounds.

Andrea had assumed that her tremendous weight gain had happened because of her lack of exercise, since her diet hadn't changed much since college. Yet she still used a treadmill for thirty minutes three or four times a

The Myth of Gastric Bypass

Gastric bypass surgery is a weight-loss surgical procedure that physically rewires the digestive system. The stomach is cut and stapled, so a remaining 2-ounce pouch limits the amount of food a person can eat at one time. The small intestine is also cut and reattached to the newly formed stomach pouch. The duodenum of the small intestine is literally bypassed.

This bypass of the first portion of the small intestine prevents the patient from absorbing all the nutrients out of the small amount of food that can still fit in the tiny pouch. As time passes, the stomach pouch stretches in size. After about a year and a half, the pouch has an 8-ounce capacity.

At about the one-and-a-half- to two-year mark after gastric bypass surgery, those with Metabolism B usually note that their weight loss abruptly stops. Right after that, they start to slowly but surely regain weight. Although the surgery bypasses the duodenum of the small intestine, it does not bypass the genes for Metabolism B. Ironically, these patients end up needing to follow the Metabolism Miracle after having permanently rewired their GI tract.

week. She had put genuine effort and time into four very popular diet approaches before giving up and deciding to go for the bypass. She was tired of dieting and gaining weight. She was tired of failing. She was tired of feeling tired. Andrea was resigned to do the surgery, deal with the possible side effects, and move on with her life.

We assessed Andrea's symptoms. Her grandmother had type 2 diabetes, and her father, who took medication for high cholesterol and high blood pressure, was recently warned to "watch his sugar." Andrea carried a good portion of her weight around her middle. She complained about being depressed and about the way she looked and felt. She had recently suffered a panic attack and cried easily. She described herself as a carb addict, craved crunchy foods and chocolate, and couldn't seem to stop eating because she never felt full. She had recently begun to drink coffee for energy.

Andrea's fasting lab data showed a blood glucose level of 101 (normal is 65–99 md/dL or 3.6–5.5 mmol/L), total cholesterol of 197 (normal is less than 200), LDL cholesterol of 130 (normal is less than 100), and "good" HDL cholesterol of 35 (normal is greater than 45). She had a history of irregular, heavy, clotty periods.

It was clear to me, given her rapid weight gain, placement of fat on her body, family history of diabetes and metabolic syndrome, symptoms, and lab work, that she had Metabolism B and could benefit hugely from the Miracle. Andrea, however, had come to my office to check off the "I met with the dietitian box" on her presurgery questionnaire.

I told Andrea that gastric bypass is a permanent rearrangement of the GI tract, but it does not bypass the genes for Metabolism B. She might lose a hundred pounds in a year, but as soon as the stomach stretches to a certain capacity (about eight ounces), carb intake can again trip up the pancreas's hyperactivity and cause weight gain. I see many patients at less than two years after this major surgery, to teach the Metabolism Miracle for weight reduction. They have had a permanent gastric bypass and end up on the very same diet they could have followed before such a drastic measure was taken.

I asked Andrea to consider giving my program a four-month chance. If, at the end of four months, she still wanted to go on with the surgery, I would understand. Andrea decided to give the Metabolism Miracle a chance, with the understanding that if it didn't work for her, I would clear her dietarily for the surgery. I planned to see her at the eight-week, twelve-week, and sixteen-week marks for follow-up, diet progression, and weigh-ins.

At eight weeks, a new Andrea appeared, looking bright, healthy, happy, and confident. She had lost twenty-one pounds of fat tissue, which gives the appearance of a forty-two-pound weight loss on traditional diets. Her new lab data was markedly improved, with glucose and cholesterol in the normal range. She was exercising by briskly walking forty-five minutes five times a week. Her clothes were loose, and she mentioned that she was hooking her bra two links smaller! She had energy, felt peaceful, and was hopeful.

We advanced her meal plan to Step Two. Andrea was hesitant about adding the required carbohydrate of Step Two because in the past, when she reintroduced carbohydrate in Phase Two of another popular low-carb diet, she regained her weight. I explained that the Miracle is devised specifically for her metabolism and that her fat loss, improved labs, and general well-being would continue. Taking a leap of faith, Andrea moved on to Step Two and returned in a month after losing seven additional pounds of fat (which looks like fourteen pounds on a traditional diet). At this point, Andrea decided to proceed with the Metabolism Miracle and put her gastric bypass plans on the back burner.

Andrea's weight loss continued, and, within a year, she hit her desired weight, with all her labs in the normal range. She lives her life on the maintenance phase of the Miracle, runs five days a week, and plans on entering a five-kilometer run this summer.

SARAH SENDS HER SCALE PACKING

Sarah is a thirty-eight-year-old woman who recently gave birth to her second child, a nine-pound girl, Caroline. She decided to return to her tried-and-true point-counting program to drop the pounds she had gained during her pregnancy. Every morning, she dutifully stepped onto her bathroom scale. (Sarah knew just how to stand on the scale to get her lowest weight!) After her previous pregnancy, when she needed to lose weight, her standby diet and exercise program easily did the trick. After Caroline's birth, she told herself, "Within a week, I'll be down about five pounds—water loss, true, but . . . at least the scale will move!!!" But this time it was different:

Monday morning: 157 pounds . . . "Day One of the 'new me'"

Tuesday morning: 157 pounds . . . "I guess it takes a few days to kick in"

Wednesday morning: 158 pounds . . . "Wait a minute, I *gained* weight?"

Thursday morning: 158.5 pounds . . . "This is ridiculous. I'm starving and gaining?"

Friday morning: 156 pounds . . . "Eureka! Progress!"

Saturday morning: 157 pounds . . . "Back to my original weight? The scale must be broken."

Sunday morning: 157.5 pounds . . . "No comment."

Monday morning: 156.5 pounds . . . "Okay, now I'm cooking."

Tuesday morning: 157 pounds . . . "@#%$! That's it!!!"

Wednesday morning: 157.5 pounds . . . "Diet over!"

After several attempts to lose weight on her original program, Sarah met with me for weight loss. Based on her symptoms, family history, and lab work, she and I discussed her trying the Miracle program. After explaining that her weight loss would always be "different than before," as it was driven by the overmetabolism of carbohydrate, I asked her to wait one month to step on the scale again. She couldn't wait. Every day she stepped on—and sure enough, at first, her weight loss had no pattern. At the end of one month, though, she had lost appreciable weight and fat, looked great, and felt great. She finally trusted that her body would respond to the program but in its own way. She now weighs herself monthly and has learned to use her body measurements, clothes size, and energy levels to mark her progress.

14

THE POWER OF POSITIVE THINKING

In a book that is meant to help you improve your health, lose weight, and enhance well-being, I would be remiss not to include a brief chapter on the power of positive thinking.

Patient after patient walks into my office depressed, frustrated, and exhausted, having lost hope about improving his or her health and weight. Initially, many have a hard time making eye contact or even smiling. I keep a box of tissues nearby because tears often flow on the first visit. The longer people have lived without help for the symptoms of Metabolism B, the more despondent they feel.

I felt exactly the same way more than twenty-five years ago, when my own Metabolism B began to manifest itself and impede my health. I was depressed, lethargic, angry, anxious, and pessimistic. I had difficulty mustering up any good feelings, let alone feeling positive about my future. I had no idea at that time, as type 2 diabetes marched forward in my body, that a hormonal imbalance had shaken up everything in my world, including the way my body used its fuel.

When you start the Metabolism Miracle program, you will learn the simple, straightforward mechanics of how best to eat with your unique metabolism, Metabolism B. I know that parts of this program seem counterintuitive. Who would have thought that you must eat right before bed? It seems wrong to have a snack before you exercise in the morning. And how can a food as healthy as lentil soup bump up your weight more than peanuts or cheese?

I know that you've seen it all when it comes to dieting, and you are tired of the disappointments after so much work. But this time around, believe that this program—this new understanding of your body and its best maintenance—will change your life in a way that you have long dreamed about. Please take a leap of faith with this program. Part of your job, as you follow the dream, is to believe that it will work.

I never used to believe that one's thoughts could influence the outcome of life. But as I watch my patients' spirits begin to lift on the first eight weeks of the Metabolism Miracle, and as I see them start to believe again in their power to control their own future, it is like watching a bird that has long been caged take flight. Your body has become your prison, but believing you can change that will help usher you toward a speedy recovery and a bright, healthy future.

I am now a firm believer that your mind, and the thoughts you let it form, very much impact the outcome of every day of your life. If you tell yourself, "It'll never work," "I will never lose this weight," and "Why bother?" you may never make it through the first three days of Step One. But when the same people who once looked for fault with everything and everyone, and lived every day feeling miserable and irritable, start to instead tell themselves, "This will work for me," "I will lose this weight and keep it off," and "I will know perfect weight and excellent health," they fortify their own conviction and make it all happen with the Miracle.

The more often you tell yourself positive thoughts, the more you will believe the words and feel the positive energy slowly but surely change the

SAY THIS . . .	INSTEAD OF THIS . . .
"I am getting thinner and healthier every day."	"I don't see anything happening."
"I am doing this very well."	"I hope I can do this."
"I feel so much more alive and energetic."	"I'm tired."
"I am a success."	"I have always failed."
"The Miracle will work for me because it was designed for me."	"I hope this works."
"I can feel my energy returning."	"I have no energy."
"My clothes are getting looser every day."	"I look heavy in this outfit."

way you see the world. Before you fall asleep at night and the very first thing in the morning, speak positively to yourself.

When you fill your mind and life with positive good thoughts, they will overflow into a positive way of living. The Metabolism Miracle starts a new beginning to your life. Expect it to work for you, know it will work for you, and watch it work for you. For the first time in a long time, you will work with your metabolism instead of against it, and you will be in tune with your body and newfound health.

PART FOUR

Recipes

BEVERAGES

CHOCOLATE–PEANUT BUTTER SMOOTHIE

For Steps One, Two, and Three;
count as 5-gram net carb (5 × 5 carb)

Serves 1

- 8 ounces cold water

- 4 ice cubes

- 1 tablespoon whipping cream

- 1 tablespoon natural smooth peanut butter

- 2 heaping tablespoons low-carb chocolate protein powder

Place all the ingredients in a blender and blend to your preferred consistency.

ORANGE DREAMSICLE SMOOTHIE

For Steps Two and Three; **1 smoothie = 1 carb serving**

Serves 1

- 8 ounces cold water

- 4 ice cubes

- 2 heaping tablespoons low-carb vanilla protein powder

- 1 peeled orange, membrane and seeds removed

Place all the ingredients in a blender and blend to your preferred consistency.

Yearning for a Vanilla, Strawberry, or Chocolate Milk Shake?

For a high-protein, extra nutritious, low-carb shake, in a blender, combine an EAS Carb Control Shake (choose your favorite flavor), 1 cup ice, and 3 tablespoons creamer.

DARK CHOCOLATE DREAMER

For Steps One, Two, and Three;   Serves 1
count as 5-gram net carb (5 × 5 carb)

  6 ounces hot brewed coffee

  ⅓ cup half-and-half or unsweetened soy milk

  ½ ounce dark chocolate, chopped

  Dollop of light whipped cream (chocolate-flavored, if preferred)

Pour the hot coffee into a mug and set aside.

Heat the half-and-half and dark chocolate together in a saucepan over low heat until melted and smooth, stirring constantly.

Pour into the coffee and serve topped with the whipped cream.

GINGER CHAI REFRESHER

For Steps One, Two, and Three; **count as no carb**   Serves 4

  4 chai tea bags

  3 cups boiling water

  Ice

  1 liter diet ginger ale

  4 cinnamon sticks, for garnish (optional)

Place the tea bags in a teapot. Pour the boiling water over the tea bags and brew for 10 minutes. Remove and discard the tea bags and let cool completely.

Add your desired quantity of ice to four beverage glasses. Pour ¾ cup of cooled tea into each glass. Top with the ginger ale and garnish each glass with a cinnamon stick.

MIRACLE MOJITO

For Steps One, Two, and Three; **count as no carb**   Serves 1

2 sprigs fresh mint

1 tablespoon lime juice

1 ounce vodka (optional)

Ice

2 ounces diet cranberry-raspberry cocktail (2 grams net carb in 8 ounces)

4 ounces seltzer

Lime slice, for garnish

Remove the mint leaves from one sprig and place in the bottom of a glass with the lime juice and vodka (if using).

Muddle the mint leaves slightly to infuse the mint flavor.

Fill a glass halfway with ice and pour in the cranberry-raspberry cocktail. Top with the seltzer.

Garnish with the rest of the mint and the slice of lime.

BREAKFASTS

VEGETABLE FRITTATA

For Steps One, Two, and Three; **count as no carb**

Cooking oil spray

1 (9- or 10-ounce) package frozen asparagus tips, or 1 cup cooked "hodgepodge" neutral veggies

1 medium yellow bell pepper, seeded and cut into strips

1 medium red bell pepper, seeded and cut into strips

1 medium onion, finely chopped

1 medium zucchini, chopped

12 eggs, beaten well, or 3 cups liquid egg substitute

½ cup half-and-half

½ cup low-fat milk

1 tablespoon chopped fresh dill

1 tablespoon chopped fresh parsley

1 teaspoon salt

½ teaspoon black pepper

1 cup shredded low-fat Cheddar cheese

Preheat the oven to 350°F. Coat an 8-inch-square or 7-by-11-inch baking pan with cooking oil spray.

Bring 4 cups of salted water to a boil in a large saucepan. Add the asparagus tips. Cover and bring to a boil, then lower the heat and simmer for 3 minutes.

Add the bell peppers and onion. Cover and bring again to a boil, then lower the heat and simmer for about 2 minutes more.

Drain the boiled veggies in a colander. Add the zucchini to the vegetable mixture and stir.

Spread the vegetable mixture evenly in the baking pan and set aside.

In a large bowl, whisk together the eggs, half-and-half, milk, dill, parsley, salt, and black pepper. Pour the egg mixture over the vegetables. Top with the cheese.

Bake uncovered for 30 to 40 minutes, or until a knife inserted in the center comes out clean.

Shortcuts to Flavorful Veggies

Use chicken broth instead of water when steaming or boiling vegetables like Brussels sprouts, broccoli, and cauliflower. This adds richness and flavor and takes the place of adding extra fat like butter or cheese.

Sprinkle grated Parmesan on top of steamed veggies to punch up their flavor without adding carbs or significant fat.

EASY EGG CUPS

For Steps One, Two, and Three;   Serves 4 (1 egg cup/serving)
count as no carb

> **Cooking oil spray**
>
> **4 ounces shredded low-fat cheese**
>
> **8 strips cooked turkey bacon, finely chopped**
>
> **4 whole eggs**
>
> **Salt and pepper**
>
> **4 tablespoons light cream**
>
> **4 tablespoons grated Parmesan cheese**

Preheat the oven to 350°F. Spray the bottom and sides of 4 cups of a muffin tin with cooking oil spray.

Drop 1 ounce of the shredded cheese into each cup.

Place one-quarter of the bacon into each cup.

Break one egg into each cup, leaving whole.

Add salt and pepper to the cream, mix well, and place 1 tablespoon in each cup.

Sprinkle the top of each cup with 1 tablespoon of the Parmesan.

Bake for 10 minutes. If desired, brown the cheese under the broiler for 2 to 3 minutes. Serve warm.

MIRACLE QUICHE

For Steps One, Two, and Three; **count as no carb**   Serves 4

Cooking oil spray

1 tablespoon butter

½ medium onion, diced

2 cups sliced mushrooms

1 cup diced fresh broccoli florets

½ cup light cream

4 ounces grated low-fat Cheddar cheese

Salt and pepper

6 eggs, beaten

Preheat the oven to 325°F. Coat the bottom and sides of a 9-inch ceramic or glass pie pan with cooking oil spray.

Melt the butter in a skillet and sauté the onion, mushrooms, and broccoli until soft.

Heat the cream in a medium saucepan until hot; do not boil. Remove from the heat and stir in the cheese until it melts.

Add the sautéed mushrooms, broccoli, salt, and pepper to the cheese mixture and let cool for 5 minutes.

Add the eggs to the mixture and mix well.

Pour into the pie pan and bake for 45 to 50 minutes, until the custard is set, or a knife inserted in the center of the quiche comes out clean. Cool on a rack for at least 5 minutes before slicing.

CRUSTLESS HAM, CHEDDAR, AND VEGGIE QUICHE

For Steps One, Two, and Three; **count as no carb**   Serves 4

Cooking oil spray

2 tablespoons butter

2 teaspoons canola oil

1 medium onion, finely chopped

½ green bell pepper, seeded and finely chopped

1 cup sliced mushrooms

6 eggs, beaten

½ cup light cream

¼ teaspoon salt

⅛ teaspoon black pepper

½ pound ham, diced into small cubes

8 ounces shredded low-fat Cheddar cheese

1 large fresh tomato, seeded and diced

10 ounces frozen chopped spinach, completely thawed, with excess liquid
  squeezed out

Preheat the oven to 350°F. Lightly coat a 10-inch pie plate or quiche dish
with cooking oil spray and set aside.

In a skillet, melt the butter and oil. Add the onion, bell pepper, and mushrooms, and sauté until the onion turns glossy and is tender; set this mixture
aside.

In the same skillet used for the sautéing, stir together the eggs, cream, salt,
and pepper, and heat for 5 minutes, stirring constantly.

In the bottom of the pie plate, distribute the diced ham, shredded Cheddar
cheese, chopped tomato, and spinach. Top with the sautéed vegetable mixture.

Pour the egg mixture over the veggie, ham, and cheese base.

Bake for approximately 50 minutes, or until a knife inserted in the center of
the quiche comes out clean. Cool on a rack for at least 5 minutes.

BANANA MUFFINS

For Steps Two and Three;
**15 grams net carb,
or one 11–20 gram carb serving**

Makes 12 (1 muffin/serving)

Cooking oil spray

1½ cups old-fashioned rolled oats

1 tablespoon baking powder

½ teaspoon baking soda

⅛ teaspoon salt

1 cup mashed bananas

2 tablespoons sucralose

¼ cup unsweetened natural applesauce

½ teaspoon vanilla extract

1 egg, beaten lightly

Preheat the oven to 350°F. Coat 12 cups of a muffin pan with cooking oil spray.

In a blender or food processor, grind the oats into a flourlike consistency. After grinding, you need 1 cup of "oat flour."

Mix together the oat flour, baking powder, baking soda, and salt.

In a small bowl, beat together the banana, egg, and sucralose. Stir in the applesauce and vanilla extract. Fold the banana mixture into the flour mixture until just combined.

Scoop the batter into the muffin cups. Fill any empty muffin cups halfway with water.

Bake for 15 to 20 minutes, or until a toothpick inserted into center of a muffin comes out clean. Let cool in the pan on a wire rack for 5 minutes, then remove from the pan and let cool on the wire rack.

FAUX BREAKFAST HASH BROWNS

For Steps One, Two, and Three; **count as no carb**   Serves 4

1 medium onion, chopped

8 slices cooked turkey bacon, chopped

1 medium head fresh cauliflower, grated

2 tablespoons olive oil (plus more as needed)

Salt and pepper

In a large skillet over medium-high heat, cook the onion and bacon until the onion is golden and the bacon is cooked. Transfer the bacon to paper towels and remove any excess fat. Chop the bacon and return it to the skillet.

Add the cauliflower and 2 tablespoons oil and stir until the cauliflower is tender and browned all over. Add oil as needed to assist in cooking.

Season to taste with salt and pepper.

Delicious Fruity Yogurt—Without the Extra Carb Grams

Change delicious plain Greek yogurt ($\frac{1}{2}$ cup = a 5 × 5 carb choice) into fruit-flavored yogurt without the added carb grams. I add a sprinkle of fruit-flavored sugar-free drink mix to my Greek yogurt, stir well, and voilà . . . I have kiwi-strawberry, lemonade, fruit punch, or even grape-flavored yogurt with no extra carb.

MIRACLE GRANOLA

For Steps One, Two, and Three;   Serves 6 (about ½ cup/serving)
count as no carb

½ **cup flaxseeds**

½ **cup sunflower seed kernels**

½ **cup unsweetened shredded coconut**

½ **cup chopped walnuts**

½ **cup chopped pecans**

½ **cup chopped almonds**

Cooking oil spray

4 tablespoons (¼ cup) butter

1 teaspoon vanilla extract

1½ **teaspoons ground cinnamon**

2 individual serving packets sucralose or stevia

Preheat the oven to 325°F.

In a medium bowl, combine the seeds, coconut, and nuts and mix well.

Lightly coat a baking sheet with cooking oil spray. Spread the mixture evenly on the baking sheet and set aside.

Melt the butter in a small saucepan and add the vanilla, cinnamon, and sweetener. Drizzle the butter mixture over the granola.

Bake for about 30 minutes, stirring every 5 minutes to avoid burning. Let cool. Store in a tightly sealed container.

A TASTE OF HOT "CEREAL"

For Steps One, Two, and Three; **count as no carb**   Serves 1

¼ cup finely chopped almonds

¼ cup finely chopped Brazil nuts

2 tablespoons ground sesame seeds

1 teaspoon butter

¼ cup light cream

⅛ teaspoon ground cinnamon

1 (1 gram) packet Splenda

Pinch of salt, if desired

In a food processor, finely process the almonds, Brazil nuts, and sesame seeds.

Place the nut mixture in a microwave-safe cereal bowl.

Add the butter, cream, cinnamon, Splenda, and salt (if desired) and mix well.

Microwave on high for 30 seconds, or until the butter is melted. Stir, close your eyes, and think "hot cereal."

SILVER DOLLAR PANCAKES

For Steps One, Two, and Three;   Serves 5 (6 pancakes per serving)
count as 5 grams net carb (5 × 5 carb)

Cooking oil spray

1 cup part-skim ricotta cheese

⅓ cup soy flour

1 tablespoon canola oil

½ teaspoon vanilla extract

1 (1 gram) packet Splenda

Pinch of salt

4 eggs, beaten

Spray a griddle pan or skillet with cooking oil spray.

In a mixing bowl, blend together the cheese, flour, oil, vanilla extract, Splenda, and salt.

Fold in the eggs and mix into a batterlike consistency.

Spoon onto the hot pan and lightly brown on both sides.

Serve with carb-free syrup, light whipped cream, or a dollop of carb-free jelly.

APPETIZERS AND SNACKS

CLAM AND CRAB DIP

For Steps One, Two, and Three;
count as no carb

Makes approximately 2½ cups of dip

1 (8-ounce) package light cream cheese

¼ cup olive oil

¼ cup light mayonnaise

1 (6½-ounce) can minced crabmeat, drained

1 (6½-ounce) can minced clams, drained

Salt and pepper

2 tablespoons finely chopped fresh dill

¼ cup finely chopped fresh parsley

¼ teaspoon garlic powder

¼ teaspoon onion powder

1 splash hot sauce

In a medium saucepan, over low heat, combine all the ingredients. Stir occasionally for 30 minutes, or until warmed thoroughly.

Transfer to a covered container and chill overnight.

Serve as a dip for "free veggies"—green or red bell pepper strips or rings, cauliflower or broccoli florets, mushroom caps, or whole green beans.

EASY PIZZA

For Steps One, Two, and Three;   Serves 1
count as 5 grams net carb (5 × 5 carb)

Cooking oil spray

1 low-carb tortilla or wrap (<5 grams net carb)

A scant ¼ cup crushed tomatoes with seasonings

Salt and pepper

Dried oregano, basil, onion powder, and/or garlic powder, if desired

½ cup shredded mozzarella cheese

Grated Parmesan cheese

Preheat the oven to 350°F. Coat a cookie sheet lightly with cooking spray.

Place the tortilla on the cookie sheet. Spoon the tomatoes evenly over the tortilla.

Sprinkle very lightly with salt, pepper, and your favorite pizza spices, such as oregano, garlic powder, onion powder, and/or garlic powder to taste.

Sprinkle evenly with the mozzarella. Top with a sprinkle of Parmesan.

Bake for 5 minutes, or until the cheese thoroughly melts.

FETA-STUFFED MUSHROOMS

For Steps One, Two, and Three;   Serves 2 (1 mushroom/serving)
count as no carb

Cooking oil spray

2 portobello mushrooms (5–6 ounces each)

Oil from the sun-dried tomatoes (below)

1 (4-ounce) package crumbled feta cheese

½ cup chopped pitted ripe olives

2 tablespoons chopped oil-packed sun-dried tomatoes

Preheat the oven to 425°F. Coat a cookie sheet with cooking oil spray.

Remove and discard the mushroom stems. Place the mushroom caps, stem side up, on the cookie sheet, brush the inside of each mushroom with oil from the sun-dried tomatoes, and set aside.

In a small mixing bowl, combine the cheese, olives, and tomatoes and mix well.

Divide the cheese mixture equally and place atop the mushrooms.

Bake for 10 minutes, or until completely heated. Serve warm.

MIRACLE GRILLED CHEESE

For Steps One, Two, and Three;
count as 5 grams net carb (5 × 5 carb)

Serves 1

Cooking oil spray

1 teaspoon butter

1 low-carb tortilla or wrap (with 5 grams or less net carb)

½ cup shredded cheese of your choice (light provolone, Cheddar, or low-fat American)

Melt the butter in a small nonstick skillet coated with cooking oil spray.

Place the tortilla on top of the butter; spread the cheese all over the tortilla.

When the tortilla bottom is golden brown and the cheese begins to melt, flip the tortilla in half to close it up.

Heat for 15 seconds on both sides. Serve warm.

STUFFED JALAPEÑOS

For Steps One, Two, and Three; **count as no carb**

Serves: 8 (3 jalapeños/serving)

24 large jalapeños

Cooking oil spray

1 pound 85–93% lean ground beef

Salt and pepper

16 ounces light cream cheese, at room temperature

1 cup shredded light Cheddar cheese

Preheat the oven to 350°F.

Cut the stems off the jalapeños and slice down one side to remove the seeds and veins. Set aside.

Coat a large skillet with cooking oil spray. Cook the ground beef over medium-high heat, breaking it apart and stirring frequently for 7 to 8 minutes, or until browned. Drain any excess fat, season with salt and pepper to taste, and let cool.

Combine the cream cheese, Cheddar, and beef in a large bowl.

Coat a cookie sheet with cooking oil spray. Stuff the mixture into the peppers, using a small spoon, and arrange the peppers on the baking sheet.

Bake for 40 to 45 minutes, or until the peppers are soft. Serve immediately.

MIRACLE GUACAMOLE

For Steps One, Two, and Three;   Makes 1 cup guacamole (½ cup/serving)
count as no carb

1 ripe avocado, halved and pitted

½ small onion, grated

1 medium ripe tomato, chopped

2 teaspoons lemon juice

1 tablespoon fresh cilantro, chopped

Hot chile sauce (optional)

Use a spoon to scoop the avocado flesh into a small bowl. Mash until soft but still a little lumpy.

Stir in the onion, tomato, lemon juice, and cilantro, plus hot sauce to taste.

Chill for 1 hour to allow the flavors to blend.

SPINACH PARTY DIP

For Steps One, Two, and Three;   Makes about 3 cups dip (½ cup/serving)
count as no carb

- **12 ounces 1% low-fat cottage cheese**

- **1 (10-ounce) package frozen chopped spinach, thawed**

- **1 (8-ounce) can water chestnuts, drained and chopped**

- **½ cup light sour cream**

- **¼ cup dried vegetable soup mix**

- **2 teaspoons grated onion**

- **¼ teaspoon salt**

Using a hand mixer or food processor, blend the cottage cheese until smooth and creamy. Transfer to a large mixing bowl.

Drain the spinach in a colander, pressing it to free its excess liquid. Wrap the spinach in paper towels and press to remove all excess liquid.

Add the spinach, water chestnuts, sour cream, soup mix, onion, and salt to the cheese; stir well.

Cover and chill for at least 2 hours. Serve with a platter of neutral veggies.

CHICKEN QUESADILLAS

For Steps One, Two, and Three;
count as 5 grams net carb (5 × 5 carb)

Serves 6 as an appetizer
(1 tortilla/serving)

Cooking oil spray

6 low-carb tortillas (with 5 grams or less net carb per tortilla)

1½ cups shredded light Cheddar cheese

1½ cups grilled chicken breast, cut into cubes

2 avocados, peeled, pitted, and chopped

¾ cup prepared salsa

½ cup light sour cream

Preheat the oven to 200°F.

Coat a heavy skillet with cooking oil spray and place over medium heat.

Lightly coat one side of a tortilla with cooking oil spray and place, oil side down, in the skillet.

Sprinkle ¼ cup of the cheese evenly over one half of the surface of the tortilla.

Top with ¼ cup of the chicken, ¼ cup of the avocado, and a heaping table-spoon of the salsa.

Fold the other half of the tortilla over the ingredients and cook for 1 to 2 minutes per side, or until the cheese melts and the tortilla is browned. Place the cooked quesadilla on a baking tray in a warm oven. Repeat with the five remaining tortillas.

Cut each tortilla into three small wedges. Serve warm with a dollop of the sour cream and the remaining salsa.

SAVORY LETTUCE BOWLS

For Steps One, Two, and Three;
count as no carb

Serves 8 as an appetizer
(2 lettuce cups/serving)

Stir-Fry Sauce

2 tablespoons cornstarch

2 tablespoons soy sauce (low-sodium, if desired)

1 tablespoon sesame or peanut oil

1 cup water

Filling

1 head Boston lettuce

1 tablespoon peanut oil

2 cloves garlic, minced

2 teaspoons minced fresh ginger

3 bell peppers (combine red, yellow, and/or green for color), seeded and chopped

1 pound 85–93% lean ground beef or lean ground turkey

To prepare the sauce, in a small bowl, whisk together the cornstarch, soy sauce, oil, and water until smooth. Set aside.

Remove eight small bowl-shaped leaves from the lettuce. Rinse, dry with towels, and set aside.

Heat the peanut oil in a large nonstick skillet over medium-high heat. Cook the garlic and ginger for 1 minute, stirring constantly. Stir in the peppers and cook for 3 minutes. Remove the peppers and set aside. In the same skillet, brown the ground beef for 8 to 10 minutes, breaking the meat apart with a fork to create a smooth consistency. Drain the fat.

Add the peppers to the browned meat. Stir in the stir-fry sauce and cook for 1 minute, or until thickened.

Spoon ⅓ cup of the beef mixture into each lettuce cup and serve.

CRISPY TORTILLA CHIPS

For Steps One, Two, and Three;   Serves 1
count as 5 grams net carb (5 × 5 carb)

- **Cooking oil spray**

- **1 low-carb tortilla (with 5 grams or less net carb)**

- **Garlic powder**

- **Salt and pepper**

- **1 tablespoon grated Parmesan cheese**

Preheat the oven to 425°F. Coat a cookie sheet with cooking oil spray.

Cut the tortilla into eight chip-size triangles. Place the triangles on the cookie sheet.

Lightly spray the tortilla triangles with cooking oil spray.

Immediately sprinkle the desired amount of garlic powder, salt, pepper, and cheese onto the triangles.

Bake for 5 to 8 minutes, or until golden brown and crispy. Watch periodically to make sure they don't burn. Let cool before eating.

Carb-Free Taco Shells

Fill crisp and crunchy lettuce leaves with your seasoned taco meat (beef or chicken), shredded cheese, chopped tomatoes, guacamole, sour cream, etc. Since everything is "neutral," go to town!

CHEESY CHIPS

Steps One, Two, and Three; **count as no carb**   Serves 1

Cooking oil spray

6 tablespoons shredded low-fat Cheddar cheese

2 tablespoons crumbled well-cooked turkey bacon, drained and blotted to reduce fat

Salsa, for dipping (optional)

Lightly coat a nonstick frying pan with cooking oil spray. Heat over medium heat until hot.

Place six mounds of the cheese (about 1 tablespoon each) on the hot pan surface, spaced well apart. Sprinkle with pepper, if desired. Sprinkle the top of each mound with bacon crumbles.

Cook for 1 minute, or until the outer edges begin turning light brown and are crispy on the bottom. Flip and crisp the other side for about 1 minute.

Remove from the pan and place on paper towels to remove any excess fat. The chips are ready to eat—and delicious with a dip of salsa!

PARMESAN CHIPS

For Steps One, Two, and Three; **count as no carb**   Serves 1

Cooking oil spray

Coarsely grated Parmesan cheese (from specialty cheese section of grocery stores)

Preheat the oven to 400°F. Coat a cookie sheet with cooking oil spray.

Spoon 1-tablespoon spoonfuls of the cheese onto the cookie sheet. Pat down each spoonful to form a little disk. Bake for 5 minutes.

Let cool before you try to remove the chips from the cookie sheet.

SWEET AND CRUNCHY NUTS

Steps One, Two, and Three; **count as no carb**   Serves 4 (½ cup/serving)

Cooking oil spray

¾ cup pecan halves

¾ cup walnut halves

½ cup whole almonds

1 egg white, lightly beaten

½ cup sucralose or stevia

½ teaspoon ground cinnamon

2 tablespoons butter

Preheat the oven to 250°F. Coat a cookie sheet with cooking oil spray.

In a medium bowl, combine the nuts. Add the egg white and toss to coat the nuts.

In a microwave-safe cup, combine the sweetener and cinnamon with the butter. Cover and microwave for 10 seconds, or until the butter is melted. Stir. Drizzle over the nuts, tossing to coat.

Spread the nut mixture evenly on the cookie sheet. Bake for 20 to 30 minutes, or until the nuts are toasted, stirring every 10 minutes. Let cool on waxed paper. Store in an airtight container.

SWEET NUT TREAT

For Steps One, Two, and Three;
count as no carb

Makes 2 cups of
sweetened walnut halves

2 tablespoons butter

2 cups walnut halves

½ cup granulated Splenda

1 tablespoon vanilla extract

2 tablespoons ground cinnamon

¼ teaspoon ground nutmeg

In a large skillet, melt the butter over medium heat. When the butter is melted, add the nuts and stir to coat with the butter.

Sprinkle with the Splenda, vanilla, cinnamon, and nutmeg, and stir well to coat the nuts.

Remove from the skillet, lay flat on a dish, and allow to cool. Store in an airtight container.

MM Trail Mix: An Anytime Snack

This easy trail mix is perfect to take to the movies as a 5 × 5 choice: Mix 1 cup each popcorn, cashews, peanuts, dry roasted edamame, and soy nuts in a zip-top bag. Happy munching!

HAM AND CREAM CHEESE "PACKETS"

For Steps One, Two, and Three; **count as no carb**

Makes approximately 16 "package" appetizers

4 ounces (half of an 8-ounce package) light cream cheese, softened

¼ cup finely chopped scallions

½ teaspoon prepared horseradish, if desired

Salt and pepper, if desired

1 pound sliced deli ham (16 slices)

Approximately 16 tiny pitted olives, for garnish

In a small mixing bowl, mix the cream cheese, scallions, horseradish, salt, and pepper.

Place a spoonful of the mixture in the center of each piece of ham.

Make a square of each ham slice by folding in the sides toward the middle.

Top the little "packet" with an olive and secure with a toothpick.

SUN-DRIED TOMATO DIP

For Steps One, Two, and Three;
count as no carb

Makes about 2½ cups of dip

- 8 ounces low-fat cottage cheese

- 8 ounces ricotta cheese

- 1 finely chopped scallion

- ½ cup finely chopped red or green bell pepper

- ¼ cup finely chopped oil-packed sun-dried tomatoes

- 1 tablespoon fresh basil or 1 teaspoon dried

- 1 teaspoon lemon juice

- ⅛ teaspoon salt

- ⅛ teaspoon black pepper

Combine all ingredients in a blender or food processor. Blend until smooth. Refrigerate for at least 2 hours.

Serve as a dip for "free veggies"—bell pepper rings, broccoli florets, celery sticks, or mushroom caps.

PEPPERONI PIZZA DIP FOR FRESH VEGGIES

For Steps One, Two, and Three;
count as no carb

Serves 5 (½ cup/serving)

8 ounces light cream cheese

½ cup light sour cream

1 teaspoon light Italian seasoning

¼ teaspoon garlic powder

½ cup seasoned crushed tomatoes

½ cup chopped turkey pepperoni

½ cup chopped red onion

½ cup seeded and chopped green bell pepper

1 cup shredded part-skim mozzarella cheese

Preheat the oven to 350°F.

In a large bowl, mix the cream cheese, sour cream, Italian seasoning, and garlic powder until smooth. Spread in a 9-inch pie pan.

Spoon the tomatoes over the cream cheese mixture. Sprinkle with the pepperoni, onion, and pepper. Bake for 10 minutes.

Remove from the oven and top with the cheese. Bake for 5 minutes more, or until the cheese is melted and the dip is heated through.

Serve with your choice of fresh crudités.

PESTO CHERRY TOMATOES

Steps One, Two, and Three;   Serves: 6 (5 tomatoes/serving)
count as no carb

30 large cherry tomatoes

¾ cup firmly packed fresh basil leaves

¾ cup firmly packed fresh flat-leaf parsley leaves

½ cup pine nuts, toasted

1 large clove garlic, quartered

⅛ teaspoon black pepper

2 tablespoons olive oil

4 ounces soft or mild goat cheese or feta cheese, crumbled (about 1 cup)

Slice the top off each tomato (about one-quarter of each tomato). Cut a thin slice off the bottom of each tomato so it stands level. Using a melon baller, scoop and discard the tomato pulp. Place the tomatoes upside down on a paper towel to drain.

To make the pesto, combine the basil, parsley, pine nuts, garlic, and pepper in a blender or food processor and blend until creamy. Add the oil and pulse until well mixed.

Transfer to a small bowl and gently stir in the cheese.

Spoon the pesto mixture into a small zippered plastic bag. Seal the bag, snip a small hole in one corner, and squeeze the pesto into the scooped-out tomatoes. Arrange the tomatoes on a serving plate. Can be served chilled or at room temperature.

Quick and Easy Recipes

- Easy 5-Gram "Pizza"

    Lightly coat a low-carb wrap with olive oil cooking oil spray. Cover the wrap with a layer of shredded mozzarella cheese. Top with seasoned crushed or diced tomatoes. Add salt, pepper, oregano, garlic powder, and basil to taste. Sprinkle with grated Parmesan or Romano cheese. Bake or broil until bubbly and the cheese is melted.

- Grilled Cheese: 5 grams net carb

    Melt a small amount of butter in a frying pan. Place a low-carb wrap in the pan and top with 2 slices of American cheese. When the bottom of the wrap is lightly browned, flip one side over the other to make a semicircle grilled cheese.

- Sandwich Wrap: 5 grams net carb

    Spread a thin coat of light ranch dressing or mayonnaise on a low-carb wrap. Fill the wrap with thinly sliced ham, turkey, and cheese. Add romaine lettuce and sliced tomato. Roll and enjoy with a dill pickle on the side.

- French Toast: 1 slice = 5 grams net carb

    Coat a nonstick frying pan with canola oil spray and heat until warm. Dip both sides of a slice of low-carb bread into a liquid of scrambled eggs or Egg Beaters. Place in the pan and lightly brown on both sides. Top with no carb/ sugar-free syrup (such as Walden Farms) and serve with a side of turkey bacon.

- Sugar-free Gelatin: zero grams net carb

    For variety, prepare a few boxes per package directions and refrigerate in separate bowls. Top with light whipped cream.

- Cauliflower Mashed Potatoes: zero grams net carb

    This can be made with fresh or frozen cauliflower. Cut up the cauliflower and boil it in chicken broth until very soft. Drain the cauliflower and put it back in the pan. Add whipped butter, shredded reduced-fat cheese, and a dollop of light sour cream. Whip or mash until you have reached the consistency of mashed potatoes. Add salt and pepper to taste.

continued on page 244

- Spaghetti Squash: zero grams net carb

     Cut a spaghetti squash in half. Place the two halves facedown on a microwave-safe dish. Cook on high for about 30 minutes. When the squash is soft to the touch, scoop out the seeds with a spoon. Using a fork, "fluff" the squash from inside. It will come out in strands like spaghetti. Sprinkle with salt as desired. Toss with marinara sauce and grated cheese for a neutral "pasta" side dish.

- Cheese Bits: zero grams net carb

     Heat a nonstick skillet and coat lightly with cooking oil spray. Drop half-dollar-size mounds of shredded Cheddar cheese into the pan. Flip when browned on one side, brown the other side, and enjoy.

- Lettuce Wraps: zero grams net carb

     Peel large leaves of lettuce to use as wraps for tuna salad or egg salad or even as taco "shells."

- Portobello Pizza Crust: zero grams net carb

     Use a portobello mushroom cap as a pizza "crust." Spread it with marinara sauce and top with shredded mozzarella cheese and your favorite neutral toppings. Broil in the toaster oven or regular oven until cheese melts and toppings are heated through.

SALADS AND SOUPS

CABBAGE SALAD

For Steps One, Two, and Three; **count as no carb**   Serves 6 to 8

- 1 medium head cabbage, finely chopped

- 1 cup light sour cream

- 2 tablespoons finely chopped fresh parsley

- ⅓ cup olive oil

- ⅓ cup light mayonnaise

- 2 tablespoons white vinegar

- ¼ teaspoon onion powder

- Salt and pepper

In a large mixing bowl, combine the cabbage, sour cream, and parsley. Distribute the sour cream over the cabbage thoroughly.

In a small bowl, whisk together the oil, mayonnaise, vinegar, onion powder, salt, and pepper. Pour the dressing over the cabbage and toss. Cover and chill before serving.

CAULIFLOWER SALAD

For Steps Two and Three;   Serves 4 (1 cup/serving)
1 cup = 1 carb serving

- 1 cup homemade (page 263) or canned chicken or vegetable broth (low-sodium, if desired)
- 10 ounces frozen cauliflower
- 10 ounces frozen peas
- ¼ cup light ranch dressing
- ¼ cup light sour cream
- ¼ teaspoon salt
- ½ teaspoon dried dill
- 1 cup peeled, diced cucumber

In a saucepan, bring the broth to a boil over medium-high heat. Add the cauliflower and peas and return to a boil. Cover and cook for 5 to 7 minutes, or until tender. Drain in a colander and let cool.

In a small bowl, whisk together the dressing, sour cream, salt, and dill.

In a medium bowl, combine the cauliflower mixture with the cucumber and dressing and toss until combined. Serve chilled.

SWEET-AND-SOUR CUKES

For Steps One, Two, and Three; **count as no carb**   Serves 6

2 cups sliced, unpeeled, well-washed cucumbers

1 cup very thinly sliced red onion

¼ cup white vinegar

¼ teaspoon dried dill

1 tablespoon powdered Splenda

Salt and pepper

Place the sliced cucumber in a medium mixing bowl and add the onion.

In a small mixing bowl, whisk together the vinegar, dill, Splenda, and salt and pepper to taste.

Pour the sauce over the cukes and chill for at least 1 hour.

Toss before serving. Serve chilled.

TENDER SPINACH SALAD

For Steps One, Two, and Three; **count as no carb**   Serves 4

10 ounces fresh baby spinach, washed and dried

1 cup fresh mushroom slices

4 hard-cooked eggs, chopped

12 slices turkey bacon, cooked and chopped

½ cup olive oil

½ cup sour cream

¼ cup red wine vinegar

½ teaspoon dry mustard

Salt and pepper

In a large bowl, toss the spinach, mushrooms, eggs, and bacon. In a separate mixing bowl, whisk together the oil, sour cream, vinegar, mustard, and salt and pepper to taste. Add the dressing to the veggies and toss to coat.

POTATO-ISH SALAD

For Steps One, Two, and Three; **count as no carb**   Serves 4 to 6

1 head cauliflower, broken into small florets

½ cup light mayonnaise

½ cup light cream

¼ teaspoon mustard (spicy preferred)

¼ teaspoon celery seeds

1 teaspoon powdered Splenda

½ onion, very finely chopped

½ green bell pepper, very finely chopped

2 hard-cooked eggs, diced, if desired

Salt and pepper

Cook the cauliflower in a large pot of boiling, salted water. Check for tenderness after 10 minutes. The cauliflower should be very soft—the texture of cooked potatoes for potato salad.

Drain and pat dry.

In a large mixing bowl, whisk together the mayo, cream, mustard, celery seeds, and Splenda.

Add the cauliflower, onion, bell peppers, and eggs to the dressing and toss lightly to coat the cauliflower.

Add salt and pepper to taste. This salad tastes best after at least 3 hours of refrigeration.

COLD PEA SALAD

For Steps Two and Three; ⅔ **cup = 1 carb serving**   Serves 4

2 cups frozen peas, thawed and dried

½ cup light sour cream

½ cup plain yogurt

¾ cup chopped scallions

Salt and pepper

Place the peas in a bowl.

In a medium mixing bowl, whisk the sour cream, yogurt, scallions, and salt and pepper to taste.

Pour the dressing over the peas and mix well. Cover and refrigerate until cold.

Serve chilled.

PASTA PRIMAVERA SALAD

For Steps Two and Three; **1 cup = 1 carb serving**   Serves 8

- **1 cup diced carrots**

- **1 cup diced yellow squash**

- **1 cup diced red onion**

- **1 cup small cauliflower florets**

- **1 cup small broccoli florets**

- **1 cup light ranch dressing**

- **2 cups cooked (½ pound dried) whole wheat pasta shapes (al dente recommended)**

- **½ cup grated Parmesan cheese**

- **1 cup diced fresh tomato**

Steam all the veggies except the tomato until crisp-tender.

Transfer to a large mixing bowl, mix with the dressing, and marinate for several hours in the refrigerator.

Mix the marinated veggies with the cooked pasta until well coated.

Add the cheese and tomato and mix thoroughly.

Serve chilled.

THREE-BEAN SALAD

For Steps Two and Three; ½ **cup = 1 carb serving**   Serves 10

1 (14-ounce) can cut green beans, drained

1 (14-ounce) can kidney beans, drained

1 (14-ounce) can chickpeas (garbanzo beans), drained

1 medium red onion, finely chopped

½ cup white vinegar

¼ cup olive oil

3 tablespoons powdered Splenda

¼ teaspoon salt

¼ teaspoon pepper

In a large mixing bowl, combine the three types of drained beans and the onions and mix well.

In a small mixing bowl, whisk together the vinegar, oil, Splenda, salt, and pepper.

Pour the dressing over the beans and mix.

Refrigerate for at least 2 hours before serving.

TURKEY WALDORF SALAD

For Steps Two and Three; **1 serving = 1 carb serving**   Serves 6

¾ cup light ranch dressing

3 tablespoons apple cider vinegar

2 level tablespoons sucralose or stevia

½ teaspoon black pepper

1 (16-ounce) bag coleslaw mix

1 (10-ounce) bag shredded carrots

1 (9-ounce) package precooked carved turkey pieces, cut into ½-inch chunks, or 9 ounces turkey breast

1 apple, cored and cut into ½-inch chunks

¾ cup chopped walnuts

In a small bowl, whisk together the ranch dressing, vinegar, sweetener, and pepper; set aside.

In a large bowl, combine the coleslaw mix, carrots, turkey, apple, and walnuts. Drizzle the salad dressing over the top and toss well to combine. Refrigerate for at least 1 hour before serving.

MY FAVORITE COBB SALAD

For Steps One, Two, and Three; **count as no carb**   Serves 4

1 head romaine lettuce, rinsed, dried, and coarsely chopped

½ head Boston lettuce, rinsed, dried, and coarsely chopped

6 slices cooked turkey bacon, crumbled

1 pound boneless, skinless chicken breast, cooked and cubed

4 hard-boiled eggs, peeled and chopped

2 tomatoes, seeded and chopped

2 ripe avocados, peeled, pitted, and cut into ½-inch cubes

2 tablespoons chopped fresh chives

⅓ cup red wine vinegar

1 tablespoon Dijon mustard

Salt and pepper

⅔ cup olive oil

½ cup blue cheese crumbles

1 to 2 teaspoons sucralose or stevia

In a large salad bowl, toss together the lettuces.

In a small skillet, cook the bacon until well browned. Drain on paper towels. Crumble the bacon and set aside.

In a shallow serving bowl, arrange the salad, placing the lettuce in the bottom and the chicken, bacon, eggs, tomatoes, and avocados in side-by-side rows over the greens. Garnish the salad with the chives.

In a small bowl, whisk together the vinegar, mustard, salt, pepper, and oil. Whisk until completely mixed. Stir in the cheese. Add the sweetener to taste, ½ teaspoon at a time. Serve the dressing separately or drizzle it over the entire salad.

SHRIMP SALAD WITH FRUIT

For Steps Two and Three; **1 serving = 1 carb serving**   Serves 4

  1 (5-ounce) package spring mix salad greens

  ½ pound cooked medium shrimp, peeled and cleaned

  1 cup canned mandarin oranges, drained

  1 ripe medium avocado, peeled, pitted, and sliced

  1 cup sliced fresh strawberries

  12 red seedless grapes, halved

  ¼ cup finely chopped Vidalia onion

  Bottled balsamic vinaigrette, as desired

On each of four plates, arrange a small bed of chilled salad greens, shrimp, orange segments, avocado, strawberries, grapes, and onion.

Drizzle with the vinaigrette and serve chilled.

MIRACLE "POTATO-LESS" SOUP

For Steps One, Two, and Three; **count as no carb**   Serves 6

- **1 head cauliflower, broken into tiny florets**

- **2 finely chopped scallions**

- **1 teaspoon finely chopped garlic**

- **4 cups chicken broth (can be low-sodium, if desired)**

- **6 strips turkey bacon**

- **4 ounces light sour cream**

- **4 ounces shredded light Cheddar cheese**

- **¼ cup butter**

- **Salt and pepper**

Gently boil the cauliflower, scallions, and garlic in the broth. After 10 to 15 minutes, check for complete tenderness of the cauliflower.

Microwave the bacon on the high setting on paper towels for 3 to 5 minutes, or until crisp. Crumble the bacon.

Remove the cauliflower from the broth (reserve the broth) and place in a mixing bowl or food processor.

Add the sour cream, cheese, and butter to the cauliflower and mix (use a hand mixer or food processor) until smooth.

Return this mixture to the broth. Add the bacon and stir over medium heat. Additional broth may be added at this time for a thinner soup.

Add salt and pepper to taste.

CORN BISQUE

For Steps Two and Three; **1 cup = 1 carb serving**   Serves 4

2 teaspoons olive oil

2 tablespoons finely chopped scallions

½ cup diced onion

¼ cup diced celery

2 tablespoons whole wheat flour

2 cups frozen corn kernels

1½ cups chicken broth

½ teaspoon Worcestershire sauce

1 drop hot sauce (optional)

½ teaspoon dried dill

½ teaspoon pepper

½ cup light cream

Heat the oil in a medium saucepan over medium-high heat.

Add the scallions, onion, and celery and stir constantly until the onion is soft and translucent.

Sprinkle the flour over the cooked veggies and stir for about 2 minutes.

Add all the remaining ingredients except the cream and heat for 10 minutes. Allow to cool slightly.

Transfer two-thirds of the veggie mixture to a blender and puree until smooth.

Add this puree to the remaining mixture and stir in the cream.

Serve warm.

ITALIAN VEGETABLE SOUP

For Steps Two and Three; **1 cup = 1 carb serving**   Serves 6 to 8

Cooking oil spray

1 pound ground mild Italian sausage, ground turkey sausage, or lean ground beef

1 cup diced onion

1 cup sliced celery

1 cup sliced carrots

1 (15-ounce) can red kidney beans, drained

1 (15-ounce) can black beans, drained

2 cups beef broth

¼ cup finely chopped fresh parsley

2 (16-ounce) cans diced tomatoes

½ teaspoon salt

¼ teaspoon oregano

¼ teaspoon basil

¼ teaspoon black pepper

2 cups shredded cabbage

Parmesan cheese, if desired

Brown the meat in a large skillet coated with cooking oil spray and drain.

Add all the ingredients except the cabbage and cheese and bring to a boil.

Lower the heat, partially cover, and simmer for 30 minutes.

Add the cabbage and simmer for another 15 minutes.

Sprinkle cheese on individual servings, if desired.

EASY FRENCH ONION SOUP

For Steps One, Two, and Three;   Serves 4 (1½ cups/serving)
count as 5 grams net carb (5 × 5 carb)

2 teaspoons olive oil

1 teaspoon butter

2 large sweet Vidalia onions, quartered and finely chopped

3 (14½-ounce) cans beef broth (low-sodium, if desired)

⅛ teaspoon black pepper

4 slices lightly buttered low-carb toast (with 5 grams or less net carb per slice)

4 ounces shredded Swiss cheese

2 teaspoons grated Parmesan cheese

In a Dutch oven or large saucepan, heat the oil and butter over medium heat until hot. Add the onions and cook for 15 to 20 minutes, stirring occasionally, until tender and browned. Stir in the broth and pepper. Bring to a boil, lower the heat to low, and simmer for 10 minutes.

Top each slice of toast with 1 ounce of Swiss and sprinkle with ½ teaspoon of Parmesan.

Microwave for 15 seconds, or until the Swiss is melted.

Place the cheese toast on the bottom of each soup bowl, ladle the onion soup over the toast, and serve immediately.

SPLIT PEA SOUP IN A HURRY

For Steps Two and Three;   Serves 8 (1 cup/serving)
1 cup = 1 carb serving

- 1 tablespoon olive oil
- 2 carrots, sliced
- 1 medium onion, finely chopped
- 2 cloves garlic, minced
- 6 cups canned chicken or vegetable broth (low-sodium, if desired)
- 1 cup dried green split peas, rinsed
- Black pepper
- 4 slices turkey bacon (optional)

Heat the oil in a Dutch oven or large pot over medium-high heat. Add the carrots, onion, and garlic. Cook, stirring, for 8 to 10 minutes, or until softened. Add the broth and split peas and bring to a boil. Lower the heat to low and simmer, partially covered, for 50 to 60 minutes, or until the vegetables are tender and the split peas have broken down. Season with pepper.

Meanwhile, cook the bacon, if using, in a small skillet over medium heat, stirring, for 3 to 5 minutes, or until crisp. Drain on paper towels and crumble into small pieces.

Ladle the soup into bowls and garnish with bacon, if desired.

HOT-AND-SOUR SOUP WITH CHICKEN

For Steps One, Two, and Three;   Serves 4 (1½ cups/serving)
count as no carb

  2 teaspoons peanut oil

  8 ounces fresh mushrooms, stems removed, caps thinly sliced

  2 cloves garlic, minced

  28 ounces homemade (page 263) or canned chicken broth (low-sodium, if desired)

  2 tablespoons rice vinegar

  2 tablespoons soy sauce

  ½ teaspoon black pepper

  8 ounces shredded cooked chicken

  2 cups bagged coleslaw mix

  1 tablespoon cornstarch

  1 scallion, thinly sliced

  1 teaspoon dark sesame oil

Pour the peanut oil into a large saucepan. Cook the mushrooms and garlic over medium heat for about 5 minutes, stirring occasionally.

Add the broth, vinegar, soy sauce, and pepper. Bring to a boil. Stir in the chicken and coleslaw mix. Return to a boil. Lower the heat and simmer uncovered for 20 minutes.

Add the cornstarch to the soup mixture and gently whisk until smooth. Simmer for 5 minutes, or until slightly thickened. Remove from the heat and stir in the sesame oil.

Sprinkle with the scallion and serve.

MINI MEATBALL SOUP

For Steps One, Two, and Three;   Serves 8 (1½ cups/serving)
count as no carb

1 pound 85–93% lean ground beef

½ pound ground pork

1 medium onion, finely chopped

2 cloves garlic, finely chopped

3 tablespoons Italian-style bread
  crumbs

1 teaspoon salt

½ teaspoon pepper

1 large egg, beaten

3 tablespoons olive oil

6 cups canned beef broth (low-
  sodium, if desired)

3 cups water

1 cup fresh spinach, washed well and
  chopped

¾ teaspoon dried oregano

½ teaspoon dried basil

¾ teaspoon dried parsley

In a large bowl, mix the meats, ¼ cup of the onion, half of the garlic, and the bread crumbs, salt, pepper, and egg. Cover and refrigerate for 1 hour (can be made the day before).

Heat 1 tablespoon of the oil in a medium stockpot over low heat. Add the remaining onion and garlic and cook, stirring frequently, for 5 to 7 minutes, or until the onion is softened and golden in color.

Add the broth, water, spinach, oregano, basil, and parsley. Bring to a boil. Lower the heat to low and simmer for 20 minutes. Strain and keep warm.

Transfer the meat mixture to a food processor and pulse about 30 seconds, or until smooth. Shape into 1-inch meatballs and set aside.

Heat the remaining 2 tablespoons oil in a large saucepan over medium-high heat. Cook the meatballs, turning frequently on all sides, until browned. Bring the broth to a simmer over medium heat. Add the meatballs and continue to simmer about 30 minutes.

LEMONY SCALLOP AND SHRIMP SOUP

Steps One, Two, and Three;   Serves: 4 (about 2 cups/serving)
count as no carb

   5 cups homemade (page 263) or canned chicken broth (low-sodium, if desired)

   ½ cup dry white wine

   2 teaspoons finely grated lemon zest

   ¼ teaspoon black pepper

   8 ounces fresh or frozen bay scallops, thawed, rinsed, and drained

   8 ounces frozen cooked and cleaned small shrimp, thawed, rinsed, and drained

   1 pound fresh asparagus spears, trimmed and cut into bite-size pieces

   1 cup sliced fresh mushrooms

   4 scallions, sliced

   1 tablespoon lemon juice

In a large saucepan, combine the broth, wine, lemon zest, and pepper. Bring to a boil.

Add the scallops, shrimp, asparagus, mushrooms, and scallions. Return to a boil. Lower the heat and simmer uncovered for 20 minutes, or until the asparagus is tender and the shrimp and scallops are opaque.

Remove from the heat. Stir in the lemon juice and serve immediately.

Cooking with Wine

Try a touch of wine in your sautéed dishes and sauces. The wine's alcohol gradually burns off, and the wine's flavor is left behind. Cooking wine tends to be salty and incorporates additional herbs and spices. It is often not the best choice in cooking because its lesser quality and flavor will not necessarily enhance your dish. Start simple with a dry white wine; try Sauvignon Blanc or Chardonnay or a bit of the wine you will later serve with your meal. Remember that the concentration of residual alcohol that remains in your dish depends on the length of time and the way in which it is cooked. For example, simmering a sauce for an hour will remove considerably more alcohol than baking a dish for 15 minutes.

CHICKEN BROTH

Steps One, Two, and Three;   Serves 8 (1 cup/serving)
count as no carb

1 (5-pound) roasting chicken, halved or cut into serving portions

1 large yellow onion, quartered

3 carrots, peeled and halved

3 stalks celery with leaves, cut into thirds

4 sprigs fresh flat-leaf parsley

4 sprigs fresh thyme

4 sprigs fresh dill

3 peeled cloves garlic, cut in half crosswise

½ teaspoon black pepper

7 chicken bouillon cubes (low-sodium, if desired)

10 cups water

In a 5- to 6-quart stockpot, combine the chicken, onion, carrots, celery, parsley, thyme, dill, garlic, pepper, and bouillon. Add the water. Simmer uncovered for 4 hours.

Lift out the chicken and let cool on a plate, then refrigerate. (The chicken can be used on salads, in chicken salad, as sandwich meat, or in soup.)

Strain the remaining contents of the pot through a colander and discard the solids. Put the broth in 2-quart containers and chill overnight. Remove the fat that has hardened and risen to the top of the broth.

Refrigerate or freeze for future use.

ENTRÉES

CHEESY BURGERS

For Steps One, Two, and Three; **count as no carb**   Serves 5

1 pound lean ground beef or lean ground turkey

¼ pound ground turkey sausage

2 cloves garlic, finely chopped

½ medium onion, finely chopped

2 eggs, beaten

Salt and pepper

1½ cups shredded Cheddar cheese

In a large mixing bowl, combine all ingredients except the cheese.

Wearing plastic gloves, hand mix the ingredients well.

Form into ten very thin patties (half the size of your normal precooked burger).

Place ¼ cup of the cheese between two patties and seal so the meat is entirely enclosing the cheese. Repeat with the remaining meat mixture and cheese.

Grill on an outdoor or indoor countertop grill, or broil, until cooked to individual preference.

BROILED TURKEY BURGERS

For Steps One, Two, and Three; **count as no carb**   Serves 4

Cooking oil spray

2 tablespoons olive oil

½ cup finely chopped green bell pepper

½ cup finely chopped celery

1 clove garlic, minced

½ cup finely chopped onion

1 pound ground turkey

2 eggs, beaten

1 teaspoon prepared mustard

Salt and pepper

Preheat the broiler. Coat a broiler pan with nonstick cooking spray.

Coat a large nonstick skillet with cooking oil spray and place over medium-high heat.

Heat the oil in the pan and add the green pepper, celery, garlic, and onion. Sauté for about 5 minutes. Set aside to cool.

In a medium mixing bowl, combine the sautéed veggies, ground turkey, eggs, mustard, salt, and pepper. Mix together until well combined. Shape into four patties.

Put the patties on the broiler pan and broil for about 5 minutes per side.

Steps Two and Three: Serve on an 11–20 gram net carb bun = 1 carb serving.

CHICKEN PAPRIKASH

For Steps One, Two, and Three; **count as no carb**   Serves 4 to 6

¼ **cup olive oil**

2 **cloves garlic, sliced**

3 **pounds skinless chicken parts (legs, thighs, breast)**

Salt and pepper

1 **small green bell pepper, chopped**

2 **tablespoons paprika**

1 **cup chicken broth, plus extra as needed for desired consistency**

½ **teaspoon onion powder**

8 **ounces mushroom caps or sliced mushrooms**

1 **cup light sour cream**

In a large saucepan, heat the oil and garlic over medium heat until the garlic browns. Remove and discard the garlic.

Sprinkle the chicken with salt and pepper on both sides.

Add the chicken, green pepper, paprika, broth, and onion powder to the saucepan and cook for 30 minutes over low heat.

Add the mushrooms. Continue to cook until the chicken is tender, about 15 more minutes, adding broth as needed to maintain the level of liquid during the cooking process.

Transfer the cooked chicken pieces to a platter.

Stir the sour cream into the saucepan that the chicken was cooked in and add enough chicken broth to make a gravylike consistency.

Pour the gravy over the chicken and serve hot.

CHICKEN MARSALA

For Steps One, Two, and Three; **count as no carb**   Serves 4

4 skinless chicken breast halves (about 1 pound)

2 tablespoons olive oil

3 cups sliced fresh mushrooms

2 cloves garlic, finely minced

$\frac{1}{4}$ teaspoon salt, plus a pinch

$\frac{1}{4}$ teaspoon black pepper

1 cup dry Marsala wine

2 scallions, thinly sliced

1 tablespoon cold water

1 teaspoon cornstarch

Place the chicken breasts between two pieces of plastic wrap or waxed paper. Using the flat side of a meat mallet, pound each to an even thickness (about $\frac{1}{4}$ inch thick). Remove the plastic wrap and set the chicken aside.

Heat 1 tablespoon of the oil in a large skillet over medium heat. When the oil is warm, add the mushrooms and garlic and cook for about 5 minutes, or until tender. Remove the mushrooms from the skillet and place in a medium bowl.

Without wiping the skillet clean, add the remaining 1 tablespoon oil and heat over medium heat until hot. Place two chicken breast halves in the skillet and sprinkle with $\frac{1}{8}$ teaspoon each of the salt and pepper. Cook over medium heat for 4 to 5 minutes per side, turning only once. Transfer the cooked chicken to dinner plates. Repeat for the remaining two chicken breast halves. Cover each plate with aluminum foil to retain warmth.

Add the wine to the drippings left in the skillet. Boil the mixture for 1 minute, scraping up the browned bits and mixing them through the sauce.

Return the mushrooms to the skillet and add the scallions. In a cup, stir together the water, cornstarch, and a pinch of salt. Add this to the skillet and cook until slightly thickened and bubbly. Cook, stirring, for 1 minute more.

Spoon the mushroom mixture over the chicken. Serve immediately.

CHICKEN STRATA

For Steps Two and Three; **1 serving = 1 carb serving**   **Serves 6**

   1 tablespoon olive oil

   2 cups trimmed and chopped fresh broccoli

   2 cups sliced fresh mushrooms

   ½ red bell pepper, seeded and chopped

   ½ yellow bell pepper, seeded and chopped

   Cooking oil spray

   3 light multigrain English muffins, torn or cut into bite-size pieces

   12 ounces cooked chicken breast, shredded

   1 cup shredded Swiss cheese

   4 eggs, beaten lightly

   1 cup nonfat or low-fat milk

   ¼ teaspoon black pepper

   ¼ teaspoon salt

Heat the oil in a large nonstick skillet over medium-high heat. Add the broccoli, mushrooms, and bell peppers and cook for about 8 minutes, or just until the vegetables are crisp-tender.

Lightly coat six individual 12-ounce casserole dishes with cooking oil spray. Divide half of the English muffin pieces among the dishes. Top with the chicken, then the broccoli mixture, and sprinkle with ½ cup of the cheese. Top with the remaining English muffin pieces.

In a medium bowl, whisk together the eggs, milk, salt, and black pepper. Pour evenly over each casserole. Using the back of a spoon, press the muffin pieces down. Sprinkle with the remaining ½ cup cheese. Cover the dishes with plastic wrap and chill for a minimum of 2 hours.

Preheat the oven to 325°F.

Bake the casseroles for 30 minutes, or until a knife inserted in centers comes out clean. Let stand for 10 minutes before serving.

CHICKEN FAJITAS

For Steps One, Two, and Three;   Serves 6 (1 fajita/serving)
count as no carb

4 boneless, skinless chicken breasts

2 tablespoons olive oil

3 tablespoons Fajita Seasoning Mix (recipe follows)

⅓ cup water

1 green bell pepper, seeded and cut into strips

1 medium onion, chopped

6 low-carb tortillas (with 5 grams or less net carb per tortilla)

1 cup mild salsa

1 cup shredded lettuce

1 cup grated or shredded low-fat Cheddar cheese

½ cup light sour cream

With kitchen scissors or a sharp knife, cut the chicken into thin strips and set aside.

Heat the oil in a large skillet over medium heat until hot. Add the chicken and cook for 8 to 10 minutes, or until the strips are cooked through.

Add the fajita seasoning, water, pepper, and onion and mix well. Simmer uncovered for about 20 minutes, or until the vegetables are tender.

Serve by spooning about ½ cup of the chicken mixture onto a tortilla and topping with some of the salsa, lettuce, and cheese and a dollop of sour cream.

FAJITA SEASONING MIX

For Steps One, Two, and Three;
count as no carb

Makes ¾ cup seasoning mix
(enough for 3 uses)

3 tablespoons cornstarch

2 tablespoons chili powder

1 tablespoon salt

1 tablespoon paprika

1 tablespoon sucralose or stevia

3 chicken bouillon cubes, crushed (low-sodium, if desired)

2 teaspoons onion powder

1 teaspoon garlic powder

½ teaspoon cayenne

¼ teaspoon crushed red-pepper flakes

In a small bowl, mix together all the ingredients.

Place the mixture in a glass or plastic container. Seal tightly and store with your other spices in a cool, dry place.

CHUNKY CHICKEN SALAD

For Steps One, Two, and Three; **count as no carb**   Serves 4

½ cup light sour cream

½ cup light mayonnaise

2 tablespoons fresh lemon juice

½ teaspoon salt

¼ teaspoon black pepper

2 cups cooked and cubed boneless, skinless chicken breast

½ green bell pepper, chopped

1 small red onion, chopped

¼ cup finely chopped fresh dill

¼ cup finely chopped fresh parsley

½ cup pitted, sliced black olives

In a medium mixing bowl, combine the sour cream, mayonnaise, lemon juice, salt, and black pepper. Blend well.

Add the chicken, bell pepper, onion, dill, parsley, and olives. Mix well.

Refrigerate for at least 1 hour prior to serving.

A Cheesy Bread Crumb Replacement

Instead of using carb-laden bread crumbs to coat chicken cutlets, eggplant, or fish, try seasoned grated Parmesan cheese. This substitute "breading" is neutral on all Steps of the Metabolism Miracle program. I usually beat three large eggs or pour ¾ cup liquid egg substitute in a small bowl. In another small bowl, mix together 1 cup grated Parmesan, ¼ teaspoon garlic powder, 1 tablespoon dried parsley flakes, ½ teaspoon Italian seasoning, and ¼ teaspoon ground black pepper. Dip each chicken cutlet into the egg bowl, shake off the excess, and then dip the cutlet on both sides into the grated cheese bowl. Continue as you would with your traditional breaded recipe.

SMOKED SAUSAGE GUMBO

For Steps One, Two, and Three;   Serves 4
count as 5-gram net carb
(eliminate carrots in Step One)

2 tablespoons olive oil

2 stalks celery, chopped

1 medium onion, chopped

1 medium green bell pepper, seeded and chopped

1 clove garlic, minced

1 medium carrot, chopped (not in Step One)

¼ cup all-purpose flour

1 cup homemade (page 263) or canned chicken broth (low-sodium, if desired)

1 pound smoked turkey sausage, cut into ½-inch pieces

1 (14½-ounce) can diced tomatoes, undrained

½ cup dry white wine

2 teaspoons dried oregano

2 teaspoons dried thyme

⅛ teaspoon cayenne

Heat the oil in a large skillet over medium heat. Sauté the celery, onion, pepper, garlic, and carrot for 10 to 12 minutes, or until tender.

Stir in the flour until blended, gradually adding the broth. Bring to a boil. Cook, stirring, for 3 minutes, or until thickened.

Transfer to a 3-quart saucepot. Stir in the sausage, tomatoes, wine, oregano, thyme, and cayenne. Cover and cook over low heat for 1½ to 2 hours to let the flavors meld.

TURKEY MELTS

For Steps Two and Three; **1 serving = 1 carb serving**   Serves 4

Cooking oil spray

4 light multigrain English muffins, split

1 pound oven-baked turkey breast (from deli, thinly sliced)

4 slices Canadian bacon

4 thick slices fresh tomato

1 cup light Alfredo sauce (jarred variety)

1 cup shredded Swiss cheese

Preheat the oven to 350°F. Lightly coat a baking sheet with cooking oil spray.

Place the English muffin tops and bottoms on the baking sheet.

Divide the turkey among the four muffin bottoms. Stack with the Canadian bacon and tomato.

Top each muffin half with 2 tablespoons of the Alfredo sauce and sprinkle with ¼ cup of the cheese.

Bake for 10 minutes, or until the stacked bottoms are heated through, the cheese is bubbly, and the tops are toasted. Place the muffin tops on the bottoms and serve warm.

Ordering at the Deli Counter

Order any of your favorite subs: ham and/or turkey, cheese, lettuce, tomatoes, onions, oil, and vinegar. Remove the roll and eat all the filling as neutral, or put the filling in your own low-carb wrap as a 5 × 5 choice.

STUFFED PEPPERS

For Steps Two and Three; **1 stuffed pepper = 1 carb serving**   Serves 4

4 medium green bell peppers

½ cup sugar-free ketchup

1 cup water

1 teaspoon Worcestershire sauce

½ pound ground turkey sausage

1 cup cooked brown rice

1 large egg, beaten

1 cup frozen corn

1 teaspoon salt

¼ teaspoon black pepper

Cooking oil spray

Preheat the oven to 350°F.

Wash the bell peppers, cut the tops off (reserve the tops), core and remove seeds, and set aside.

In a small mixing bowl, whisk together the ketchup, water, and Worcestershire sauce, and set aside.

In a large bowl, stir together the sausage, rice, egg, corn, salt, and black pepper.

Put one-quarter of the mixture in each pepper. Replace the top of each pepper.

Coat a baking dish with cooking oil spray and place the filled peppers in the dish. Pour the ketchup mixture over the stuffed peppers.

Bake for 45 minutes.

MIRACLE "SPAGHETTI"

For Steps One, Two, and Three; **count as no carb**   Serves 4 to 6

1 spaghetti squash

Cooking oil spray

1 pound lean ground turkey or lean ground beef

2 cloves garlic, minced

½ cup chopped onion

½ cup chopped green bell pepper

2 (14-ounce) cans crushed tomatoes with basil and herbs

½ cup white wine

1 cup grated Parmesan cheese

Cut the squash in half and remove the seeds.

Place, facedown, in a microwave-safe dish with a ½-inch depth of water on the bottom.

Cover with plastic wrap. Make a few slits in the plastic wrap for ventilation.

Microwave on high for 10 to 20 minutes, or until tender, turning occasionally.

Coat a large skillet with cooking oil spray and place over medium heat. Add the ground turkey, garlic, onion, and pepper and brown for about 10 minutes, or until the meat is cooked.

When the meat is cooked, add the tomatoes and wine and simmer for about 30 minutes.

After the squash is cooked and has cooled enough to handle, use a fork to pull/shred it into a large bowl. It will actually look like strands of spaghetti!

Divide the spaghetti among four to six plates, top with the meat sauce, and sprinkle with the cheese.

SHISH KEBAB

For Steps One, Two, and Three; **count as no carb**   Serves 4 to 6

¼ cup olive oil

½ cup Italian dressing

2 tablespoons lemon juice

3 large cloves garlic, crushed

¼ cup white wine

¼ teaspoon salt

¼ teaspoon pepper

¼ teaspoon dried oregano

¼ teaspoon dried rosemary

1½ pounds leg of lamb or London broil, cubed for kebabs

1 large green bell pepper, seeded and cut into 8 chunks

1 large red bell pepper, seeded and cut into 8 chunks

1 large red onion, cut into 8 chunks

12 medium mushroom caps

In medium mixing bowl, combine the oil, dressing, lemon juice, garlic, wine, and seasonings.

Pour the marinade over the lamb cubes and stir to completely coat. Cover tightly and refrigerate for 24 hours, occasionally stirring the sauce over the lamb.

The next day, preheat the broiler.

Remove the lamb cubes from the marinade (reserve the marinade) and thread on skewers to contain only lamb. Other skewers should be used separately to create bell pepper kebabs, onion kebabs, and mushroom kebabs, as they will all be grilled for different amounts of time.

Place the shish kebabs on a broiling tray. Baste all with the marinade.

Broil about 6 inches from the heat source: the lamb skewers for 10 minutes, the bell pepper and the onion skewers for 4 minutes, and the mushroom skewers for 3 minutes.

Remove the meat and veggies from the skewers and set aside to cool enough to be handled.

Rethread a skewer with a cube of cooked lamb, then a piece of bell pepper, a piece of onion, and a mushroom, and repeat until all the ingredients have been used on as many skewers as will hold them.

Baste all the shish kebabs with the marinade.

Return the skewers to the broiler, turning frequently, until the meat is totally cooked. (Safety note: Because the marinade has been used for raw meat, be sure to cook through at high heat before serving.)

Take Off Your Coat

You may use any cooking method for proteins, except those that depend upon coating the meat or fish with flour, bread crumbs, sweetened sauces, gravies, or sweet marinades.

Grilling, baking, roasting, sautéing, and broiling all pass muster with the Metabolism Miracle plan. For additional flavoring, use carb-free spices or seasonings, such as mustard, vinegar, and garlic. Citrus and wine can also be used in cooking.

GINGER FLANK STEAK

For Steps One, Two, and Three; **count as no carb**   Serves 4

  1½ pounds flank steak, trimmed of excess fat

  1 cup canned beef broth (low-sodium, if desired)

  ¼ cup hoisin sauce

  3 tablespoons soy sauce (low-sodium, if desired)

  2 scallions, sliced

  ¼ cup white wine

  1 tablespoon sucralose or stevia

  1 teaspoon grated fresh ginger

  3 cloves garlic, minced

  Cooking oil spray

Place the steak in a zippered plastic bag and set in a shallow dish.

To make the marinade, whisk together the broth, hoisin sauce, soy sauce, scallions, wine, sweetener, ginger, and garlic in a small bowl.

Pour the marinade over the steak in the bag and seal it. Refrigerate for at least 4 hours, turning the bag occasionally. The marinated steak can then be broiled or grilled.

To broil: Preheat the broiler.

Drain the steak and discard the marinade.

Lightly coat the unheated rack of a broiler pan with cooking oil spray. Position the rack 5 inches from the heat source. Place the steak on the rack and broil for 15 to 18 minutes, turning once, until medium done (160°F).

To serve, thinly slice the steak across the grain.

To grill: Coat the grill rack with cooking oil spray before lighting it. Ignite the grill.

Drain the steak and discard the marinade.

When the coals are medium hot, place the steak directly on the rack and grill uncovered for 17 to 20 minutes, turning once, until medium done (160°F).

To serve, thinly slice the steak across the grain.

PHILLY STEAK AND CHEESE

For Steps One, Two, and Three; **count as no carb**   Serves 4

Cooking oil spray

1 pound "minute"/wafer steaks (beef or chicken)

2 green bell peppers, cored and sliced in 1-inch slices

1 large onion, diced

2 cloves garlic, finely chopped

½ cup beef or chicken broth

1 cup shredded provolone cheese

Preheat the oven to 350°F. Coat a large skillet and a shallow baking pan with cooking oil spray.

Break the steaks into quarters and quickly brown in the skillet. Drain off the excess fat and place the steak in the baking pan.

In the hot skillet, over medium-high heat, sauté the pepper, onion, and garlic until golden brown. Spoon the sautéed veggies on top of the steak.

Pour the broth over the steak and veggies.

Bake, uncovered, for 20 minutes.

Top with the cheese and broil for 3 minutes, or until the cheese gets bubbly.

Step One: Serve inside a low-carb wrap (<5 grams of net carb) = 5 × 5 carb.

Steps Two and Three: Serve in a warm 11–20 gram net carb bun = 1 carb serving.

MEDITERRANEAN MEAT LOAF

For Steps One, Two, and Three;   Serves 8 (two ½-inch slices/serving)
count as 5-gram net carb (5 × 5 carb)

1 (12-ounce) jar roasted red peppers, drained and chopped

4 slices low-carb bread (with 5 grams or less net carb per slice), torn into small pieces

2 eggs, slightly beaten

¼ cup chopped fresh basil

¼ cup chopped fresh parsley

½ teaspoon salt

½ teaspoon black pepper

½ teaspoon garlic powder

1 cup marinara sauce (no-sugar-added variety)

2 pounds lean ground beef

Preheat the oven to 350°F.

In a large bowl, combine the red peppers, bread, eggs, basil, parsley, salt, pepper, garlic powder, and ¾ cup of the marinara sauce in a large bowl. Mix well.

Add the ground beef and knead well until thoroughly blended. (Wear plastic gloves, if desired.)

Lightly pat the beef mixture into a 9-by-5-inch loaf pan. Spoon the remaining ¼ cup marinara sauce over the meat loaf.

Bake uncovered for 1¼ to 1½ hours, or until a meat thermometer inserted in the center registers 160°F.

Remove from the oven and let the pan stand on a wire rack for 15 minutes.

Drain the fat from the pan. Loosen the meat loaf from the sides of the pan. Carefully remove the meat loaf and slice to serve.

SWEDISH MEATBALLS

For Steps One, Two, and Three; **count as no carb**

Serves 4 (7 meatballs/serving)

1 pound lean ground beef

1 medium onion, finely chopped

1 medium green bell pepper, seeded and finely chopped

2 cloves garlic, finely chopped

¼ cup finely chopped fresh dill

¼ cup finely chopped fresh parsley

½ teaspoon Italian seasoning

¼ teaspoon grated nutmeg

1 teaspoon dried dill

1 large egg, beaten

½ teaspoon salt

Black pepper

Cooking oil spray

2 tablespoons olive oil

¾ cup beef broth

¼ cup white wine

In a large mixing bowl, combine the ground beef, onion, green pepper, garlic, fresh dill, parsley, spices, egg, salt, and pepper.

Wearing plastic gloves, use your hands to mix the ingredients evenly.

Form into about thirty 1-inch mini meatballs.

Coat a nonstick skillet with cooking spray and add the oil. Heat over medium heat.

Cook the meatballs, in batches if necessary, shaking the skillet occasionally, until they are browned on all sides and cooked through. Remove the meatballs from the skillet and place on paper towels, to drain excess grease.

Add the broth and wine to the skillet and cover. Turn up the heat and cook over high heat for about 3 minutes.

Add the meatballs back to the pan and cook in the sauce for 10 minutes, spooning the sauce over the meatballs as it thickens.

Serve immediately.

SLOW-COOKED BEEF AND BEAN CHILI

For Steps Two and Three; **count as 1 cup = 1 carb serving**   Serves 8

1 (14-ounce) can diced tomatoes, undrained

1 (14-ounce) can chopped tomatoes and green chile peppers, undrained

1 cup vegetable juice cocktail or tomato juice

1 cup beef broth

1 tablespoon chili powder

1 teaspoon ground cumin

1 teaspoon dried oregano

3 cloves garlic, peeled and minced

2 pounds boneless beef chuck roast, cut into 1-inch cubes

2 large onions, chopped

3 stalks celery, chopped

1 large green bell pepper, seeded and chopped

1 (15-ounce can) kidney beans, drained

1 (15-ounce can) chickpeas (garbanzo beans), drained

In a 6-quart slow cooker (such as a Crock-Pot), combine the diced and chopped tomatoes, vegetable juice, broth, chili powder, cumin, oregano, garlic, beef, onions, celery, and pepper.

Cover and cook on the low heat setting for 8 to 10 hours, or on the high heat setting for 4 to 5 hours.

Stir in the kidney beans and chickpeas.

Cook on the high setting for 15 minutes longer.

VEAL OR BEEF STROGANOFF

For Steps One, Two, and Three; **count as no carb**   Serves 4

Cooking oil spray

1½ pounds veal, cubed, or sirloin steak, sliced

2 tablespoons olive oil

2 green bell peppers, seeded and chopped

1 large onion, chopped

Salt

1 tablespoon finely chopped fresh basil

1 pint light sour cream

1 tablespoon whole wheat flour

Black pepper

Coat a nonstick skillet with cooking oil spray. Add the veal cubes or steak and brown for 10 to 12 minutes. Remove from the skillet and set aside.

Pour the oil into the skillet. Add the bell peppers and onion. Sauté over medium heat until tender, stirring constantly, for 7 to 9 minutes.

Add the browned veal or steak to the skillet. Add enough water to cover the veal, along with salt to taste and the basil. Simmer over medium heat for 20 to 30 minutes, or until tender.

Add the sour cream, flour, and black pepper. Stir well. Keep simmering until the sauce thickens.

Remove from the heat. Serve over steamed green beans or soy noodles to keep it neutral or over the appropriate amount of whole wheat noodles for Step Two or Three.

BROKEN NOODLES

For Steps Two and Three; **1 cup = 1 carb serving**   Serves 6

8 ounces ground turkey sausage

8 ounces 85–93% lean ground beef

1 medium onion, chopped

2 cloves garlic, minced

2 cups marinara sauce (no-sugar-added variety)

1 cup water

8 ounces whole-grain lasagna-type noodles, broken into pieces

2 cups chopped zucchini

1 cup part-skim ricotta cheese

¼ cup grated Parmesan cheese

1 tablespoon chopped fresh parsley

½ teaspoon salt

¼ teaspoon black pepper

1 cup shredded part-skim mozzarella cheese

In a large skillet over medium heat, brown the sausage, ground beef, onion, and garlic. Break the beef apart with a fork while cooking to remove any lumps. Drain off the fat, keeping the meat mixture in the skillet.

Add the marinara sauce and water. Mix well. Bring to a boil, stirring occasionally. Add the noodles and zucchini. Return to a boil.

Lower the heat and simmer, partially covered, for 12 to 14 minutes, or until the noodles are tender, stirring occasionally.

Meanwhile, in a small bowl, combine the ricotta, Parmesan, parsley, salt, and pepper. Using a spoon, drop the cheese mixture into six mounds over the mixture in the skillet. Sprinkle the mozzarella over the top.

Cover and cook over low heat for 5 minutes, or until the cheese mixture is heated through.

Let stand, uncovered, for 5 minutes before serving so that the cheese can set.

GLAZED HAM

For Steps One, Two, and Three; **count as no carb**

Makes about 2½ servings per pound of ham

1 tablespoon all-purpose flour

Precooked ham (shank portion)

Whole cloves

Dijon mustard

½ cup Splenda brown sugar

Preheat the oven to 325°F.

Place the flour in a large (14-by-20-inch or 19-by-23-inch) oven bag. Place the oven bag in a baking dish large enough to hold the ham.

Score the ham by making ¼-inch diagonal cuts in a diamond pattern. Insert one clove in the center of each diamond.

Place the ham inside the bag, fat side up. Close the bag with a twist tie. Pierce the top of the bag with six to eight small slits.

Bake the ham for 12 minutes per pound, minus 30 minutes (see next step).

Thirty minutes before it is done, remove the ham from the oven. Increase the oven temperature to 375°F. Slit the bag down the center and open to the sides to completely expose the ham.

Brush the entire top of ham with the mustard. Sprinkle with the brown sugar.

Bake for an additional 30 minutes at 375°F.

GRILLED PORK KEBABS

For Steps One, Two, and Three; **count as no carb**   Serves 8

1 pound pork tenderloin, cut into ½-inch cubes

¼ cup bottled Italian dressing (low-fat preferred)

¼ cup white wine

2 cloves garlic, minced

1 teaspoon dried oregano

¼ teaspoon salt

½ teaspoon black pepper

8 (6-inch long) wooden skewers, soaked in warm water for at least 1 hour

24 grape tomatoes

24 small mushrooms

24 pearl onions, peeled

Olive oil cooking spray

Combine the cubed pork, dressing, wine, garlic, oregano, salt, and pepper in a zippered plastic bag placed inside a shallow dish. Seal the bag and refrigerate for at least 2 hours or even overnight.

Thread the pork cubes onto the skewers, alternating with the tomatoes, mushrooms, and onions. Lightly coat the filled skewers with olive oil cooking spray.

Heat your grill to medium hot. Place the skewers on the grill and cook for 15 to 18 minutes, turning frequently, until the pork is cooked through.

SLOW-COOKED LAMB WITH WILD RICE

For Steps Two and Three; **1 cup = 1 carb serving**   Serves 6

Cooking oil spray

2 pounds boneless lamb shoulder roast

2 tablespoons olive oil

1 cup vegetable or tomato juice

1½ cups beef broth

1 cup uncooked wild rice

1 teaspoon curry powder

½ teaspoon salt

¼ teaspoon pepper

2 medium carrots, diced

2 stalks celery, diced

1 small onion, diced

Salt and pepper

Have ready a 4-quart slow cooker.

In a large nonstick skillet coated with cooking oil spray, brown the meat on all sides in the oil.

In the slow cooker, combine the vegetable juice, broth, rice, curry powder, salt, carrots, celery, onion, salt, and pepper.

Place the roast in the cooker.

Cover and cook on the low heat setting for 8 to 9 hours, or on the high heat setting for 4 to 4½ hours.

SEAFOOD DELIGHT

For Steps One, Two, and Three; **count as no carb**   Serves 4 to 6

¼ cup butter

¼ cup olive oil

¼ cup white wine

2 teaspoons crushed garlic

Cooking oil spray

½ pound flounder fillet

1 pound large sea scallops

1 pound whole jumbo shrimp

2 tablespoons finely chopped fresh parsley

¼ cup grated Parmesan cheese (optional)

Preheat the oven to 400°F.

Melt the butter in a small saucepan over medium heat, then add the oil, wine, and garlic. Heat until the garlic is lightly browned, then remove and discard the garlic. Set the sauce aside.

Coat a glass baking dish with cooking oil spray. Cut the flounder into six pieces. Arrange the flounder, scallops, and shrimp in the baking dish.

Pour the sauce over the fish and sprinkle with the parsley.

Bake, uncovered, until the fish is flaky and thoroughly cooked.

Sprinkle with the cheese, if desired, and serve.

EGGPLANT ROLLATINI

For Steps One, Two, and Three; **count as no carb**   Serves 6

3 medium eggplant, cut lengthwise into ¼-inch slices

Salt

Cooking oil spray

Olive oil

2 cups part-skim ricotta cheese

1 large egg, beaten

1 cup shredded mozzarella cheese

½ cup grated Parmesan cheese

¼ cup finely chopped fresh parsley

2 cups seasoned crushed tomatoes or your own marinara sauce, made without
added tomato paste or tomato sauce

Preheat the oven to 350°F.

Lightly sprinkle both sides of the eggplant with salt. Place the eggplant
slices in a colander in the sink for about 15 minutes. Rinse and blot dry the
eggplant.

Heat a large sauté pan coated with cooking oil spray over medium heat. Add
about 2 tablespoons oil.

Add the eggplant in batches and cook until soft and pliable, replacing the oil
as needed. Transfer the eggplant to a platter.

In a large mixing bowl, mix the ricotta, egg, mozzarella, Parmesan, and
parsley.

Coat a glass baking dish with cooking oil spray.

One eggplant slice at a time, spread the cheese mixture over an entire slice
and then roll up. Place the roll, seam side down, in the baking dish.

After all the eggplant is rolled, pour the marinara sauce over the rolls and top
with a little more Parmesan, if desired.

Bake for 30 minutes and serve.

PASTA-FREE VEGGIE LASAGNA

For Steps One, Two, and Three; **count as no carb**   Serves 12

Cooking oil spray

1 large or 2 small eggplant, cut lengthwise into ½-inch slices

2 pounds part-skim ricotta cheese

4 cloves garlic, chopped

¼ cup grated Parmesan cheese

2 cups shredded part-skim mozzarella (reserve ½ cup for the top layer)

1 bunch fresh basil, chopped

1 tablespoon Italian seasoning

Salt and pepper

1 small onion, chopped

1 medium bell pepper (red, yellow, or orange), seeded and chopped

4 cups sliced mushrooms

1 bunch broccoli, florets only, coarsely chopped

3 ounces fresh spinach, chopped

2 cups crushed tomatoes or your own marinara recipe, made with no added
    tomato paste or tomato sauce

3 small zucchini, cut lengthwise into ⅛-inch slices

3 small yellow squash, cut lengthwise into ⅛-inch slices

Preheat the oven to 350°F. Coat a baking sheet with cooking oil spray.

Arrange the eggplant on the baking sheet and bake for 15 to 20 minutes, or
until flexible but not completely cooked.

In a mixing bowl, mix the ricotta with half of the garlic. Stir in the Parmesan and $1\frac{1}{2}$ cups of the mozzarella, the basil, Italian seasoning, salt, and pepper and set aside.

In a large nonstick skillet coated with cooking spray, sauté the onion, bell pepper, mushrooms, broccoli, and remaining garlic for about 5 minutes. Add the spinach and remove from the heat. Allow to cool, and then add to the cheese mixture.

To assemble, spread a thin layer of the tomatoes in a large baking dish, such as a 3-quart Pyrex lasagne dish, then layer:

Eggplant slices

Ricotta mixture

Zucchini slices

Squash slices

Crushed tomatoes

Eggplant slices

Ricotta mixture

Zucchini or squash slices

Crushed tomatoes

Ricotta mixture, and so on

Layer until you run out of ingredients! End with a layer of zucchini or eggplant and top with tomatoes or sauce. Sprinkle with the reserved $\frac{1}{2}$ cup mozzarella.

Bake for 1 to $1\frac{1}{2}$ hours, until hot and bubbly.

SPINACH FETA PIE

For Steps One, Two, and Three; **count as no carb**   Serves 6

Cooking oil spray

2 (10-ounce) packages frozen chopped spinach, thawed

1 large onion, chopped

3 cloves garlic, minced

1 tablespoon olive oil

1 cup low-fat cottage cheese, drained

4 ounces feta cheese, crumbled

2 large eggs, beaten lightly with 2 tablespoons milk

1 teaspoon Italian seasoning

¼ teaspoon black pepper

½ cup grated Parmesan cheese

1 tablespoon butter, at room temperature

Preheat the oven to 350°F. Lightly coat a 9-inch pie plate with cooking oil spray.

Place the spinach in a colander and squeeze out any excess water. Transfer the spinach to layered paper towels and press out any remaining water. Set aside.

In a medium saucepan over medium heat, cook the onion and garlic in the oil for about 8 minutes, or until translucent.

Stir the reserved spinach, cottage cheese, feta, eggs, and seasonings into the onion mixture. Mix well.

Spoon the mixture into the pie plate. Sprinkle with the Parmesan and dot with the butter.

Bake uncovered for 30 to 35 minutes, or until a knife inserted near the center comes out clean. To serve, cut into six wedges.

VEGETARIAN POTLUCK

For Steps Two and Three;   Serves 4 or 5 (1½ cups/serving)
1½ cups = 1 carb serving

   5 cups homemade or canned vegetable broth (low-sodium, if desired)

   3 cloves garlic, peeled

   2 teaspoons olive oil

   1 medium onion, chopped

   6 ounces shiitake mushrooms, stemmed, wiped clean, and sliced

   1 small head bok choy (¾ pound) cut into ½-inch pieces, stems and greens
      separated

   3½ ounces Chinese wheat noodles

   1 (14- to 16-ounce) package firm tofu, drained, patted dry, and cut into ½-inch
      cubes

   1 cup grated carrots

   1 tablespoon rice vinegar

   2 teaspoons soy sauce (low-sodium, if desired)

   1 teaspoon toasted sesame oil

   ¼ cup chopped scallions, for garnish

In a Dutch oven, combine the broth and garlic and bring to a boil. Lower the
heat to medium-low and let simmer, partially covered, for 20 minutes. Discard the garlic.

Meanwhile, heat the olive oil in a large nonstick skillet over medium-high
heat. Add the onion and cook for about 5 minutes. Add the mushrooms and
continue to cook for another 5 minutes. Add the bok choy stems and cook,
stirring often, for about 5 minutes, or until tender.

Add the mushroom mixture to the broth. Add the noodles, lower the heat to
medium-low, and simmer for 3 minutes. Add the bok choy greens and tofu.
Simmer for about 3 minutes, or until heated through. Stir in the carrots,
vinegar to taste, soy sauce, and sesame oil.

Serve garnished with the scallions.

TOFU AND VEGGIES

For Steps One, Two, and Three;   Serves 4 (1 cup/serving)
count as no carb

  2 tablespoons olive oil

  1 medium onion, chopped

  2 cloves garlic, minced

  1 (14- to 16-ounce) extra-firm tofu, rinsed, drained, blotted dry, and cut into
    bite-size pieces

  1 cup cooked spinach, chopped and squeezed dry

  1 cup crushed tomatoes, drained

  ¼ teaspoon salt

  ¼ teaspoon black pepper

  ½ cup Parmesan cheese

Heat the oil in a large skillet over medium-high heat. Add the onion and garlic. Cook, stirring, until golden brown.

Add the tofu and brown lightly on both sides, turning once. When the tofu is golden brown, add the spinach, tomatoes, salt, pepper, and cheese. Cover and bring to a boil, lower the heat, and simmer for 5 minutes, stirring occasionally.

MUSHROOM-CHEESE "BURGERS"

For Steps One, Two, and Three; **count as no carb**   Serves 4

   4 portobello mushrooms

   2 tablespoons olive oil

   Salt and pepper

   1 teaspoon Italian seasoning, crushed

   4 slices provolone cheese

Preheat grill.

With a sharp knife, scrape the gills from mushroom caps.

Drizzle the mushrooms with the oil. Sprinkle with the salt, pepper, and Italian seasoning.

Cook the mushrooms on the rack of an uncovered charcoal grill, directly over medium-hot coals, for 6 to 8 minutes, turning halfway through cooking.

Top each mushroom with a cheese slice.

WHITE BEAN–STUFFED TOMATOES

For Steps Two and Three; **1 cup = 1 carb serving**   Serves 4

4 large red tomatoes

1½ cups soft bread crumbs (from whole wheat bread)

1 (15-ounce) can white kidney beans (cannellini beans), drained and rinsed

½ cup grated Parmesan cheese

1 teaspoon Italian seasoning

1 tablespoon olive oil

2 cloves garlic, minced

⅛ teaspoon salt

⅛ teaspoon black pepper

Cooking oil spray

1 tablespoon butter, melted

Preheat the oven to 350°F.

Slice off ¾ inch from the top of each tomato. Finely chop the tomato tops to produce about ¾ cup of chopped tomato and set aside.

Using a melon baller or a spoon, remove and discard the seeds from each tomato. Put the hollowed-out tomatoes upside down on paper towels to drain.

In a large bowl, stir together the chopped tomato, ¾ cup of the bread crumbs, all the beans, ¼ cup of the cheese, ¾ teaspoon of the Italian seasoning, salt, and pepper.

Spoon the bean mixture into the hollowed-out tomatoes.

Place the stuffed tomatoes in a 2-quart square baking dish lightly coated with cooking oil spray.

In a small bowl, stir together the remaining ¾ cup bread crumbs, ¼ cup cheese, and ¼ teaspoon Italian seasoning. Sprinkle evenly over the tomatoes and drizzle with the butter.

Bake uncovered for 20 to 30 minutes, or until the bread crumbs are golden brown and the tomatoes are heated through.

SIDE DISHES

NOT YOUR MOM'S GREEN BEAN SIDE DISH

For Steps One, Two, and Three;
count as no carb

- 1½ pounds fresh green beans, trimmed and cut into bite-size pieces
- 1 tablespoon olive oil
- 6 ounces sliced fresh mushrooms
- 4 shallots, chopped
- 3 cloves garlic, finely minced
- 2 teaspoons chopped fresh thyme
- ½ teaspoon salt
- 1 (2.8-ounce) can French-fried onions

Add the green beans to a large pot of boiling, salted water. Cook for 10 minutes, or until tender, and drain in a colander.

Meanwhile, heat 2 teaspoons of the oil in a large nonstick skillet over medium-high heat. Add the mushrooms and shallots, stirring occasionally, for about 5 minutes, or just until tender. Add the garlic, thyme, and salt. Cook, stirring constantly, for about 2 minutes, or until fragrant. Stir in the green beans and heat through.

To make the topping, heat the remaining 1 teaspoon oil in a small nonstick skillet over medium heat. Add the French-fried onions and cook, stirring occasionally, for 1 to 2 minutes, or until lightly toasted.

Transfer the beans to a large bowl, sprinkle with the French-fried onions, and serve immediately.

BROCCOLI-CHEESE CASSEROLE

For Steps One, Two, and Three; **count as no carb**   Serves 4

2 cups reduced-fat shredded Cheddar cheese

2 cups sliced mushrooms

1 cup chopped scallions

½ cup light cream

¼ cup olive oil

½ teaspoon salt

2 cups chopped fresh broccoli

Cooking oil spray

Preheat the oven to 350°F.

In a medium saucepan over low heat, combine all the ingredients. Cook for 5 minutes, stirring constantly.

Coat a 2-quart casserole dish with cooking oil spray. When the cheese melts, spoon the mixture into the dish.

Bake for 30 minutes.

Serve warm.

BROCCOLI WITH CHEESE SAUCE

For Steps One, Two, and Three; **count as no carb**   Serves 4

   1½ pounds fresh broccoli, cut into florets

   ¾ cup homemade (page 263) or canned chicken or vegetable broth
     (low-sodium, if desired)

   ⅓ cup light sour cream

   ½ cup shredded low-fat Cheddar cheese

   2 teaspoons lemon juice

   2 teaspoons Dijon mustard

Place the broccoli and broth in a large microwave-safe bowl. Cover and microwave on high for 5 to 6 minutes, or until fork-tender. Drain, reserving ½ cup broth, and keep warm.

For the sauce, combine the sour cream, cheese, reserved broth, lemon juice, and mustard in a small microwave-safe bowl. Whisk until smooth. Cover and microwave on high for 2 to 3 minutes, or until warmed. Serve over the broccoli.

ROASTED SWEET POTATO "FRIES"

For Steps Two and Three;   Serves 4
½ potato = 1 carb serving

Cooking oil spray

1 pound sweet potatoes

½ teaspoon salt

½ teaspoon garlic powder

½ teaspoon onion powder

¼ teaspoon black pepper

Pinch of ground nutmeg

Preheat the oven to 425°F. Lightly coat a 9-by-13-inch baking pan or cookie sheet with cooking oil spray.

Scrub the sweet potatoes. Slice them lengthwise into quarters and cut each quarter in half. Set aside.

In a small bowl, combine the salt, garlic powder, onion powder, and nutmeg and place in a large zippered plastic bag.

Coat the sweet potato wedges with cooking oil spray. Add the wedges to the bag and shake until all pieces are coated with the seasoning mix.

Arrange the seasoned sweet potato wedges in a single layer on the baking pan.

Bake for 30 to 35 minutes, or until brown and tender, turning once during the baking.

HERBED MASHED PARSNIPS

For Steps Two and Three; ¾ **cup = 1 carb serving**   Serves 4

2 pounds parsnips, peeled and cut into 2-inch pieces

½ teaspoon dried chives

½ teaspoon dried parsley

½ teaspoon dried dill

¾ cup half-and-half

2 tablespoons butter

Salt and pepper

Bring a large pot of salted water to a boil. Add the parsnips and cook for 15 to 18 minutes, or until tender when pierced with a fork.

Drain the parsnips in a colander and return them to the pot. Add the chives, parsley, and dill.

Mash the parsnips with a potato masher or hand mixer, leaving them rather rough. Stir in the half-and-half and butter. Mash until the parsnips reach your desired texture. Season to taste with salt and pepper.

SWEET POTATO LATKES

For Steps Two and Three;   Serves 3 (3 latkes/serving)
1 serving = 1 carb serving

1 slice low-carb bread (with 5 grams or less net carb)

1 medium sweet potato

½ medium sweet onion (such as Vidalia)

1 egg white, lightly beaten

⅛ teaspoon baking powder

⅛ teaspoon salt

Black pepper

Olive oil cooking spray

¼ cup light sour cream (optional)

Toast the bread until dark in tone. On a handheld grater, grate the toasted bread into crumbs and set aside.

Grate the sweet potato and onion. Place in a medium bowl. Stir in the egg white, bread crumbs, baking powder, salt, and pepper to taste.

Coat a nonstick skillet with olive oil cooking spray and preheat over medium heat. Drop ¼ cup of the potato mixture at a time into the skillet. Flatten the pancake with a fork or the back of a spatula. Cook for 5 to 6 minutes per side, turning only once when golden brown on the bottom. Coat the bottom of the pan with more cooking oil spray before you flip each pancake.

Serve immediately, accompanied by a dollop of sour cream, if desired.

BROWN RICE PILAF

For Steps Two and Three; ⅔ **cup = 1 carb serving**   Serves 4

1 cup uncooked brown rice

2 cups homemade (page 263) or canned chicken broth (low-sodium, if desired)

1 cup sliced mushrooms

½ cup shredded carrots

¼ cup thinly sliced scallions

¼ teaspoon black pepper

¼ teaspoon dried marjoram, crushed

1 tablespoon finely chopped fresh parsley

1 tablespoon butter

Rinse the rice in a strainer under cold running water for 30 seconds, swirling the rice around with your hand.

Pour the rice into a large bowl of water and let soak for 60 minutes to soften. Strain in a colander.

Meanwhile, bring the broth to a boil in a large pot over high heat. When the broth boils, add the mushrooms, carrots, scallions, pepper, marjoram, parsley, and butter. Return the broth to a boil. Add the rice, stirring once.

When the broth returns to a full boil, lower the heat to medium-low, cover tightly with a lid, and cook for about 40 minutes. Do not stir the rice.

After 40 minutes, remove the rice from the heat and let stand, covered, for 10 minutes.

Uncover the rice and fluff with a fork before serving.

WINTER SQUASH SOUFFLÉ

For Steps Two and Three; **1 serving = 1 carb serving**   Serves 4

Cooking oil spray

All-purpose flour

2 (12-ounce) packages frozen winter squash

4 eggs

¼ cup butter, melted

2 tablespoons Splenda brown sugar

½ teaspoon salt

⅛ teaspoon ground nutmeg

⅛ teaspoon ground cinnamon

Coat a 1½-quart soufflé dish with cooking oil spray and lightly sprinkle it with flour.

Prepare the squash according to the package directions. When cooked, drain in a colander and place in a large mixing bowl.

Meanwhile, separate the eggs, placing the yolks in a small bowl and the whites in a large bowl. Let the eggs and squash stand at room temperature for about 30 minutes.

Preheat the oven to 350°F.

In a large bowl, using a hand mixer, combine the egg yolks, squash, butter, Splenda brown sugar, salt, nutmeg, and cinnamon.

Using a hand mixer (with clean beaters), beat the egg whites separately until stiff peaks form.

With a spatula, gently stir one-quarter of the beaten whites into the squash mixture until no white streaks remain. Gently fold in the remaining whites just until incorporated.

Transfer to the soufflé dish. Bake for 55 to 60 minutes, or until the top is puffed and the center appears set. Serve immediately.

ASPARAGUS WITH GOAT CHEESE

For Steps One, Two, and Three;   Serves 4 (4 to 6 spears/serving)
count as no carb

   Cooking oil spray

   2 tablespoons pine nuts

   2 tablespoons olive oil

   1 pound asparagus spears, ends removed

   ⅛ teaspoon salt

   ⅛ teaspoon black pepper

   ¼ cup crumbled goat cheese

Coat a large skillet with cooking oil spray.

Toast the pine nuts in a small, dry skillet over medium-high heat, stirring constantly, for about 2 minutes. Set aside.

Pour the oil in the skillet and turn up the heat to medium. When the oil is hot, place the asparagus spears in the skillet. Sprinkle with the salt and pepper. Sauté the asparagus on all sides until crisp-tender, turning occasionally.

Arrange the asparagus spears on a warmed serving plate. Sprinkle the goat cheese over all and top with toasted pine nuts. Serve immediately.

CAULIFLOWER "RICE"

For Steps One, Two, and Three;   **Makes 1 head of cauliflower "rice"**
count as no carb

1 head fresh cauliflower

Salt

Using a food processor or even a hand grater, grate or chop the cauliflower until it is the size of rice (use a plain steel blade or shredder blade).

Add a sprinkling of salt to taste and microwave on high in a covered dish for 4 minutes. Do not add water. To keep it fluffy, just let the moisture in the cauliflower do its work.

Tomato Tip

Think of tomatoes as a cross between a fruit and a vegetable. Like many fruits, they have a certain amount of carbohydrate and, for that reason, you should limit them during Step One to a half cup per meal.

Most commercial or prepared tomato sauce is not allowed during Step One because it contains added sugar or concentrated paste. Consider making a quick marinara sauce of crushed tomatoes, garlic, onions, wine, and olive oil. A half-cup serving of this sauce is permitted on Step One as a 5 × 5 carb choice. Use it on steamed vegetables or as a sauce for chicken or fish.

MASHED CAULIFLOWER

For Steps One, Two, and Three; **count as no carb**   Serves 4

1 head cauliflower, florets only

2 cloves garlic, finely chopped

1 (14-ounce) can chicken broth

½ teaspoon salt

¼ teaspoon pepper

1 tablespoon butter

¼ cup light sour cream

½ cup reduced-fat shredded Cheddar cheese

Salt and pepper

In a medium saucepan over medium high heat, bring the cauliflower, garlic, broth, and salt to a boil.

Reduce the heat to medium and simmer until extremely tender.

Drain, reserving the broth.

Place the cauliflower in a blender with the pepper, butter, sour cream, and cheese. Puree, adding broth as needed for a mashed-potato consistency. Season with salt and pepper to taste.

Serve warm as you would mashed potatoes.

ZUCCHINI AND ONIONS

For Steps One, Two, and Three; **count as no carb**   Serves 4

Cooking oil spray

1 tablespoon olive oil

3 large zucchini, peeled and cut into ½-inch slices

1 medium onion, finely chopped

½ cup chopped walnuts

¼ teaspoon grated nutmeg

¼ teaspoon dried dill

Salt and pepper

Coat a large skillet with cooking oil spray. Add the olive oil and heat over medium heat.

Add the zucchini and onions and cook, stirring occasionally, for 10 minutes, or until tender.

Add the walnuts, nutmeg, dill, and salt and pepper to taste. Stir and cook for an additional minute.

Serve warm.

Succulent Side Dish: Zucchini "Fettuccine" Alfredo

Peel a zucchini and discard the outer skin. Continue peeling fettuccine-shaped strips until you reach the seeded middle of the squash. Heat 2 tablespoons olive oil in a skillet over medium heat. Add zucchini "fettucine." When softly cooked, place on your dinner plate and top with ¼ cup of jarred Alfredo sauce (make sure carb content is under 5 grams). Serve as a delicious side dish with any entrée.

SWEET POTATO FRIES

For Steps Two and Three; **eight ¼-inch fries = 1 carb serving**   Serves 4

Cooking oil spray (for pan)

2 sweet potatoes, peeled and cut lengthwise in ¼-inch strips

Olive oil cooking spray (for potatoes)

Salt and pepper

1 teaspoon ground cinnamon

2 tablespoons powdered Splenda

Preheat the oven to 450°F. Coat a cookie sheet with cooking oil spray.

Arrange the sweet potatoes on the cookie sheet. Do not overlap. Spray the potatoes with the olive oil cooking spray and sprinkle with salt and pepper.

Bake, turning every 10 minutes, for 30 to 45 minutes, or until tender. When done, sprinkle with the cinnamon and Splenda. Serve warm.

TABBOULEH

For Steps Two and Three; ½ cup = 1 carb serving   Serves 6

1 cup uncooked bulgur

2 cups boiling water

⅓ cup lemon juice

½ teaspoon salt

¼ teaspoon black pepper

2 cloves garlic, minced

3 medium tomatoes, seeded and chopped

1 cup finely chopped parsley

1 cup finely chopped scallions

½ cup finely chopped mint leaves

In a bowl, combine the bulgur and boiling water and let soak for 1 hour.

In a large mixing bowl, combine the lemon juice, salt, pepper, and garlic.

Drain the bulgur and add to the lemon juice mixture. Add the other ingredients and mix thoroughly.

Cover tightly and refrigerate for at least 1 hour.

Serve chilled.

BAKED TREATS AND OTHER SWEETS

BAKED APPLES

For Steps Two and Three; **1 filled apple = 1 carb serving**   Serves 4

Cooking oil spray

4 tablespoons butter, softened

4 tablespoons powdered Splenda

½ teaspoon ground cinnamon

½ teaspoon grated nutmeg

½ teaspoon ground allspice

4 large baking apples (such as Empire, Cortland, Golden Delicious, or Winesap), washed and cored

Preheat the oven to 350°F. Coat a baking dish with cooking oil spray.

In a small mixing bowl, blend the butter, Splenda, and spices.

Divide evenly and spoon inside the apples.

Place the filled apples in the baking dish.

Bake for 30 minutes, or until the apples are tender.

Serve warm.

CHOCOLATE BROWNIE MUFFINS

For Steps One, Two, and Three;   Makes 20 to 24 muffins
1 muffin = 5 × 5 carb

5 ounces unsweetened baking chocolate

2 cups powdered Splenda

1¾ cups soy flour

1½ teaspoons baking powder

1½ teaspoons baking soda

1 teaspoon salt

2 eggs

1 (16-ounce container) light sour cream (or use just 8 ounces for a less moist muffin)

½ cup canola oil

2 teaspoons vanilla extract

1 cup boiling water

½ cup finely chopped walnuts, if desired

Preheat the oven to 350°F. Line 20 to 24 muffin cups with cupcake liners.

Microwave the chocolate on high for about 2 minutes, or until it melts. Cover while microwaving to avoid spattering.

Combine the dry ingredients in a mixing bowl. Add the eggs, melted chocolate, sour cream, oil, and vanilla. Stir in the nuts. Slowly add the boiling water while mixing to a smooth batter. The batter will be thin.

Fill each muffin cup two-thirds full. Bake for 22 to 25 minutes.

Cool on a wire cooling rack.

These muffins are great for freezing in freezer bags and pulling out as needed. They can be topped with light whipped cream. This is a 5 × 5 carb, so wait 5 hours before having another 5 × 5 carb.

"GILDED" CINNAMON MUFFINS

For Steps One, Two, and Three;
each muffin = 5 × 5 carb

Makes 24 muffins

4 cups soy flour

1½ teaspoons baking soda

1½ teaspoons baking powder

1 teaspoon salt

5 teaspoons ground cinnamon

4 eggs

½ cup canola oil

1½ cups granulated Splenda

1 (16-ounce) container light sour cream

Preheat the oven to 350°F.

Coat 24 muffin cups with cooking oil spray or line with cupcake liners.

In a large mixing bowl, stir the soy flour, baking soda, baking powder, salt, and cinnamon.

In a separate bowl, beat the eggs and blend with the oil and Splenda. Mix together for about 30 seconds.

Add the egg mixture to the dry mixture and blend in the sour cream.

Pour the batter into the muffin cups.

Bake for 25 minutes, or until lightly browned.

Cool on a cooling rack.

ZUCCHINI MUFFINS

For Steps One, Two, and Three;   **Makes 20 to 24 muffins**
1 muffin = 5 × 5 carb

4 cups soy flour

⅓ cup ground flaxseed

1½ teaspoons baking soda

1½ teaspoons baking powder

1 teaspoon salt

1½ teaspoons ground cinnamon

4 eggs

¾ cup vegetable oil (could be ½ cup)

1½ cups sugar substitute, such as Splenda (could be less to taste)

2 medium zucchini, shredded (about 2 cups)

1 cup light sour cream

1 cup walnut pieces (optional)

Preheat the oven to 350°F.

Coat 24 muffin cups with cooking oil spray or line with cupcake liners.

In a large bowl, whisk together the soy flour, flaxseed, baking soda, baking powder, salt, and cinnamon.

In a separate bowl, mix the eggs, oil, and sugar substitute for 30 seconds, or until the sugar substitute is dissolved. Stir in the zucchini.

Stir the egg mixture into the flour mixture. Stir in the sour cream and then the walnuts, if using. Pour the batter into the muffin pan, filling the cups three-quarters full. If all 24 cups will not be used, fill the empty cups with a few tablespoons of water.

Bake for 23 to 25 minutes, or until crowned and lightly browned.

CINNAMON RICOTTA PUDDING

For Steps One, Two, and Three; **count as no carb**   Serves 1

½ cup part-skim ricotta cheese

1 tablespoon low-fat sour cream

¼ teaspoon vanilla extract

¼ teaspoon ground cinnamon

1 (1 gram) packet Splenda

Light whipped cream

In a dessert bowl, mix together the ricotta, sour cream, vanilla extract, cinnamon, and Splenda. Chill and top with light whipped cream before serving.

CHOCOLATE RICOTTA PUDDING

For Steps One, Two, and Three; **count as no carb**   Serves 1

½ cup part-skim ricotta cheese

1 tablespoon low-fat sour cream

½ teaspoon unsweetened cocoa powder

¼ teaspoon vanilla extract

1 (1 gram) packet Splenda

Light whipped cream

In a dessert bowl, mix together the ricotta, sour cream, cocoa powder, vanilla extract, and Splenda. Chill and top with light whipped cream before serving.

LEMON RICOTTA PUDDING

For Steps One, Two, and Three; **count as no carb**   Serves 1

½ cup part-skim ricotta cheese

1 tablespoon low-fat sour cream

¼ teaspoon grated lemon zest

¼ teaspoon vanilla extract

1 (1 gram) packet Splenda

Light whipped cream

In a dessert bowl, mix together the ricotta, sour cream, lemon zest, vanilla extract, and Splenda. Chill and top with light whipped cream before serving.

COOL AND CREAMY GELATIN MOUSSE

For Steps One, Two, and Three;   Makes about 8 servings (½ cup each)
count as no carb

1 (4-serving) package sugar-free gelatin, your choice of flavor

1 (8-ounce) container light cream cheese, softened

½ cup light sour cream

1 cup light whipping cream

2 teaspoons powdered Splenda

In a large mixing bowl, prepare the gelatin as directed on the box. Refrigerate for about 1 hour 15 minutes, or until almost set but still a little soft.

With an electric mixer, beat the gelatin until creamy.

While continuing to beat, add the cream cheese and sour cream and mix thoroughly.

In another bowl, whip together whipping cream and Splenda until peaks form. Gently fold into the gelatin mixture, leaving it with a marbled look— don't keep stirring until it becomes uniform in color.

Spoon into dessert dishes and chill for at least 2 hours.

NANCY'S FANCY CHOCOLATE MERINGUE COOKIES

For Steps One, Two, and Three;
3 cookies = 5 × 5 carb

Makes approximately 30 cookies

5 egg whites

¼ **teaspoon vinegar**

1½ **teaspoons vanilla extract**

½ **cup granulated Splenda**

¼ **cup Splenda Sugar Blend for Baking**

¼ **cup unsweetened cocoa powder**

¼ **cup ground pecans (optional)**

Preheat the oven to 250°F. Line several cookie sheets with aluminum foil.

Whip the egg whites until frothy. Add the vinegar and vanilla extract. Slowly add both kinds of Splenda. Beat until stiff.

Gently fold in the cocoa powder. Fold in the pecans, if using.

Using a tablespoon, drop spoonfuls of the mixture 1 inch apart on the cookie sheets.

Bake for 2 hours.

Let cool, and then peel gently from the foil. Store in an airtight container.

CHOCOLATE CUPCAKES

For Steps One, Two, and Three; **count as no carb**   Makes 6 cupcakes

5 eggs, separated

⅛ teaspoon cream of tartar

6 tablespoons butter, at room temperature

1 teaspoon vanilla extract

1 cup sucralose

2 cups almond flour

2 teaspoons baking powder

5 tablespoons unsweetened cocoa flour

Light whipped cream, for topping (optional)

Preheat the oven to 325°F. Line six cups of a muffin tin with paper or foil liners.

In a mixing bowl, whisk the egg whites and cream of tartar until stiff. Set aside.

In a separate bowl, with clean beaters, cream the butter and egg yolks until light yellow and fluffy. Add the vanilla extract and sweetener. Beat until mixed.

Add about one-third of beaten egg whites to the egg yolk mixture and mix gently. Fold the mixture into the remaining egg whites.

Fold in 1 cup of the almond flour. Gently but thoroughly fold in the remaining almond flour, the baking powder, and the cocoa, being careful not to break down the egg whites.

Fill the lined muffin tins about half full. Fill any empty muffin cups halfway with water. Bake for 15 to 20 minutes, or until the tops begin to crack. Remove from the oven and let stand for 5 minutes before removing the cupcakes from the tin. Let cool on a rack.

The cupcakes can be topped with light whipped cream immediately prior to serving.

Fat Loss Expectations on Steps One and Two

The following tables (one for men and one for women) are based on gender, height, and starting weight at the beginning of the eight-week period in Step One or Two. Remember, the Metabolism Miracle is a "fat loss" program. The weight lost is composed primarily of fat—light, voluminous tissue. A high percentage of fat loss allows for a very visual weight loss. Ten pounds of fat loss on the Metabolism Miracle will look like twenty pounds of weight loss on traditional calorie-burning diets. This is because traditional diets produce weight loss made up of water weight, muscle loss, and fat loss.

A guideline to ascertain that you are losing mainly fat is to retake your body measurements. At the end of the eight weeks, tally the total inches you've lost. Your pounds lost (plus or minus one) should equal your inches lost!

Example: Lynn loses 10 pounds after eight weeks of Step One. As she is a five-foot-three-inch woman who started the program weighing 175 pounds, the table shows that she lost between 6 and 13 pounds—right on track. Lynn then does her eight-week remeasure and sees that she lost eleven inches.

−1 ← 10 pounds → +1

A ten-pound weight loss for Lynn should come with a nine- to eleven-inch loss . . . and it did! Lynn is doing very well regarding pounds of fat lost, as indicated by number of inches lost.

WOMEN

Find your height and starting weight below to identify the number of "fat" pounds that you are expected to lose during the upcoming eight weeks on Steps One or Two. Remember, you will look like you have lost twice as much weight.

4'10"

90–130 lb = 3–5 lb fat loss	170–210 = 14–21 lb fat loss
130–170 = 6–13 lb fat loss	210–250 = 22–29 lb fat loss

4'11"

95–135 lb = 3–5 lb fat loss	175–215 lb = 14–21 lb fat loss
135–175 lb = 6–13 lb fat loss	215–255 lb = 22–29 lb fat loss

5'0"

100–140 lb = 3–5 lb fat loss	180–220 lb = 14–21 lb fat loss
140–180 lb = 6–13 lb fat loss	220–260 lb = 22–29 lb fat loss

5'1"

105–145 lb = 3–5 lb fat loss	185–225 lb = 14–21 lb fat loss
145–185 lb = 6–13 lb fat loss	225–265 lb = 22–29 lb fat loss

5'2"

110–150 lb = 3–5 lb fat loss	190–230 lb = 14–21 lb fat loss
150–190 lb = 6–13 lb fat loss	230–270 lb = 22–29 lb fat loss

5'3"

115–155 lb = 3–5 lb fat loss	195–235 lb = 14–21 lb fat loss
155–195 lb = 6–13 lb fat loss	235–275 lb = 22–29 lb fat loss

5'4"

120–160 lb = 3–5 lb fat loss	200–240 lb = 14–21 lb fat loss
160–200 lb = 6–13 lb fat loss	240–280 lb = 22–29 lb fat loss

5'5"

125–165 lb = 3–5 lb fat loss	205–245 lb = 14–21 lb fat loss
165–205 lb = 6–13 lb fat loss	245–285 lb = 22–29 lb fat loss

5'6"

130–170 lb = 3–5 lb fat loss	210–250 lb = 14–21 lb fat loss
170–210 lb = 6–13 lb fat loss	250–290 lb = 22–29 lb fat loss

5'7"

135–175 lb = 3–5 lb fat loss	215–255 lb = 14–21 lb fat loss
175–215 lb = 6–13 lb fat loss	255–295 lb = 22–29 lb fat loss

5'8"

140–180 lb = 3–5 lb fat loss	220–260 lb = 14–21 lb fat loss
180–220 lb = 6–13 lb fat loss	260–300 lb = 22–29 lb fat loss

5'9"

145–185 lb = 3–5 lb fat loss	225–265 lb = 14–21 lb fat loss
185–225 lb = 6–13 lb fat loss	265–305 lb = 22–29 lb fat loss

5'10"

150–190 lb = 3–5 lb fat loss	230–270 lb = 14–21 lb fat loss
190–230 lb = 6–13 lb fat loss	270–310 lb = 22–29 lb fat loss

5'11"

155–195 lb = 3–5 lb fat loss	235–275 lb = 14–21 lb fat loss
195–235 lb = 6–13 lb fat loss	275–315 lb = 22–29 lb fat loss

6'0"

160–200 lb = 3–5 lb fat loss	240–280 lb = 14–21 lb fat loss
200–240 lb = 6–13 lb fat loss	280–320 lb = 22–29 lb fat loss

MEN

Find your height and starting weight below to identify the number of "fat" pounds that you are expected to lose during the upcoming eight weeks on Steps One or Two. Remember, you will look like you have lost twice as much weight.

5'0"

106–146 lb = 3–5 lb fat loss	186–226 lb = 14–21 lb fat loss
146–186 lb = 6–13 lb fat loss	226–266 lb = 22–29 lb fat loss

5'1"

112–152 lb = 3–5 lb fat loss	192–232 lb = 14–21 lb fat loss
152–192 lb = 6–13 lb fat loss	232–272 lb = 22–29 lb fat loss

5'2"

118–158 lb = 3–5 lb fat loss	198–238 lb = 14–21 lb fat loss
158–198 lb = 6–13 lb fat loss	238–278 lb = 22–29 lb fat loss

5'3"

124–164 lb = 3–5 lb fat loss	204–244 lb = 14–21 lb fat loss
164–204 lb = 6–13 lb fat loss	244–284 lb = 22–29 lb fat loss

5'4"

130–170 lb = 3–5 lb fat loss	210–250 lb = 14–21 lb fat loss
170–210 lb = 6–13 lb fat loss	250–290 lb = 22–29 lb fat loss

5'5"

136–176 lb = 3–5 lb fat loss	216–256 lb = 14–21 lb fat loss
176–216 lb = 6–13 lb fat loss	256–296 lb = 22–29 lb fat loss

5'6"

142–182 lb = 3–5 lb fat loss	222–262 lb = 14–21 lb fat loss
182–222 lb = 6–13 lb fat loss	262–302 lb = 22–29 lb fat loss

5'7"

148–188 lb = 3–5 lb fat loss	228–268 lb = 14–21 lb fat loss
188–228 lb = 6–13 lb fat loss	268–308 lb = 22–29 lb fat loss

5'8"

154–194 lb = 3–5 lb fat loss	234–274 lb = 14–21 lb fat loss
194–234 lb = 6–13 lb fat loss	274–314 lb = 22–29 lb fat loss

5'9"

160–200 lb = 3–5 lb fat loss	240–280 lb = 14–21 lb fat loss
200–240 lb = 6–13 lb fat loss	280–320 lb = 22–29 lb fat loss

5'10"

166–206 lb = 3–5 lb fat loss	246–286 lb = 14–21 lb fat loss
206–246 lb = 6–13 lb fat loss	286–326 lb = 22–29 lb fat loss

5'11"

172–212 lb = 3–5 lb fat loss	252–292 lb = 14–21 lb fat loss
212–252 lb = 6–13 lb fat loss	292–332 lb = 22–29 lb fat loss

6'0"

178–218 lb = 3–5 lb fat loss	258–298 lb = 14–21 lb fat loss
218–258 lb = 6–13 lb fat loss	298–338 lb = 22–29 lb fat loss

6'1"

184–224 lb = 3–5 lb fat loss	264–304 lb = 14–21 lb fat loss
224–264 lb = 6–13 lb fat loss	304–344 lb = 22–29 lb fat loss

6'2"

190–230 lb = 3–5 lb fat loss	270–310 = 14–21 lb fat loss
230–270 lb = 6–13 lb fat loss	310–350 lb = 22–29 lb fat loss

6'3"

196–236 lb = 3–5 lb fat loss	276–316 lb = 14–21 lb fat loss
236–276 lb = 6–13 lb fat loss	316–356 lb = 22–29 lb fat loss

6'4"

202–242 lb = 3–5 lb fat loss	282–322 lb = 14–21 lb fat loss
242–282 lb = 6–13 lb fat loss	322–363 lb = 22=29 lb fat loss

6'5"

208–248 lb = 3–5 lb fat loss	288–328 lb = 14–21 lb fat loss
248–288 lb = 6–13 lb fat loss	328–368 lb = 22=29 lb fat loss

6'6"

214–254 lb = 3–5 lb fat loss	294–334 lb = 14–21 lb fat loss
254–294 lb = 6–13 lb fat loss	334–374 lb = 22–29 lb fat loss

Anxiety, Panic Disorder: Many patients with Metabolism B report feelings of anxiety and nervousness that come and go. Some describe anxiety to the point of panic attacks that can cause shortness of breath, pounding or rapid heartbeat, cold sweats, dizziness, fainting, and shakiness. Although panic attacks exist for many reasons, there is definitely a relationship between panic attacks and blood sugar fluctuations. Treatment for blood sugar panic attacks would require stabilizing the blood sugar.

Attention Deficit Disorder or Attention-Deficit/Hyperactivity Disorder: ADD/ADHD is a neurobehavioral disorder affecting between 3 and 5 percent of children under the age of nineteen. Although it typically presents itself during childhood, it can last into adulthood. This disorder is usually treated by a combination of medications, behavior and lifestyle modifications, and counseling. Interestingly, many of the symptoms of ADD/ADHD are also the symptoms of progressing Metabolism B. It seems prudent to check the fasting blood glucose of children diagnosed with ADD/ADHD to see if changes in diet might help.

Blood Glucose: Also known as blood sugar, blood glucose is the body's fuel. The amount of glucose in the blood varies throughout the day and is hormonally regulated by the pancreas. Normal blood sugar is 65–140 mg/dL (3.6–7.8 mmol/L). Blood glucose can be stored in the muscles and liver as glycogen, and excesses are stored as fat. Rises in blood glucose trigger the release of insulin. Drops in blood glucose trigger the release of glucagon.

Carbohydrate: A major nutrient found in many foods such as fruit, bread, legumes, milk, potatoes, rice, and pasta as well as sweets, desserts, and chips, carbohydrate converts 100 percent into blood glucose and is the body's preferred fuel source.

Chronic Fatigue: Also known as chronic fatigue syndrome, this type of exhaustion is an all-encompassing, draining fatigue. The person wakes up tired and remains drained throughout much of the day, making everyday life a real effort. People use the terms "washed out" or "totally drained" to describe this exhaustion. If Metabolism B is playing a part in chronic fatigue syndrome, then the hormonal balance that the Miracle provides will help alleviate this problem.

Depression (Mild): Depression is a physical medical condition involving an imbalance of brain chemicals. It is diagnosed not by a blood test but by the symptoms that the patient relates to the physician or therapist.

When a person's glucose level has sharp peaks and valleys, it causes many of the same symptoms that chemical depression causes. Because the symptoms sound so similar, the depression related to blood sugar imbalance is often misdiagnosed as chemical depression and is incorrectly treated with antidepressant medications. These patients often report little or no improvement even after the physician has changed the type or dose of antidepressant. Unfortunately, it is not commonly accepted that blood sugar imbalance can mimic the symptoms of brain chemical imbalance. It is probably prudent to check a patient's blood glucose level as part of a medical evaluation for depression. If fasting blood glucose exceeds 90 mg/dL (5 mmol/L), the Metabolism Miracle should be used (perhaps in tandem with medication for depression).

Diabetes

Prediabetes: Also known as borderline diabetes, prediabetes is a reversible condition. The diagnosis, made when fasting blood glucose is 100–125 mg/dL (5.6–6.9 mmol/L), is often considered a red flag that the patient is on the road to type 2 diabetes. With proper diet, exercise, and stress reduction, a diagnosis of type 2 diabetes may be prevented or forestalled. In an effort to be proactive, the Metabolism Miracle sets the red flag of prediabetes at 90–125 mg/dL (5–6.9 mmol/L).

Type 2 Diabetes: Type 2 diabetes, also known as adult onset diabetes, is the most common form of diabetes and is caused by either the pancreas not producing enough insulin and/or the insulin no longer fitting cells effectively (insulin resistance). Insulin is necessary for the body to use glucose for energy. It is the "key" that opens the cells so that they can accept the glucose from the bloodstream. If the pancreas does not produce enough insulin, or if the insulin can't open the cells appropriately, glucose has nowhere to go and subsequently builds up in the bloodstream. Type 2 diabetes is diagnosed with two fasting blood glucose tests over 125 mg/dL (6.9 mmol/L). Recurrent elevations of blood sugar can, over time, damage blood vessels and nerves, leading to irreversible complications involving the eyes, nerves, kidneys, blood vessels, and circulation.

Type 1 Diabetes: This is an autoimmune disease that results in the permanent destruction of insulin-producing beta cells in the pancreas. Its exact cause is unknown, but there appears to be a genetic link that may be precipitated by a virus or environmental trigger. Previously known as juvenile diabetes, its onset is usually abrupt. It is often diagnosed in children and young adults, but it can occur at any age. It results in the absence of insulin, and people with type 1 diabetes currently require insulin administration for life.

Gestational Diabetes Mellitus (GDM): GDM occurs in a pregnant woman who has never had diabetes but develops high blood glucose during the pregnancy because normal placental hormones block the action of the mother's insulin. The pancreas fails to produce adequate insulin to bring the mother's blood glucose into normal range during the pregnancy. The treatment for GDM is diet modification, exercise as directed, and, in some cases, insulin injection. Most glucose levels normalize very soon after delivery. Babies born to mothers with untreated gestational diabetes often weigh 9 pounds or more.

Gestational diabetes is routinely screened between weeks 24 and 28 of the pregnancy. Approximately 6 percent of pregnant women develop GDM. Women with a history of GDM have a greater chance of a recurrence during future pregnancies and a greater chance of developing type 2 diabetes in the future.

Fasting Blood Glucose: Fasting blood glucose is determined by a lab test drawn first thing in the morning after at least eight hours without food or calorie-containing beverages. This test can be used to determine blood glucose conditions including prediabetes or type 2 diabetes. The American Diabetes Association normal fasting blood glucose level = 65–99 mg/dL (3.6–5.5 mmol/L). Prediabetes = 100–125 mg/dL (5.6–6.9 mmol/L) (inclusive). Diabetes = *greater than or equal to* 126 mg/dL (7 mmol/L). The diagnosis of diabetes should be confirmed with a second fasting blood glucose result *greater than or equal to* 126 mg/dL.

Fat Cells: The number of fat cells you will carry throughout life is determined in utero and can again increase at the beginning of puberty. When an adult gains weight, it is the size and not the number of fat cells that increases.

Fibromyalgia: This constellation of symptoms includes fatigue, muscle pain, and stiffness. It also often includes constipation, headaches, decreased short-term memory, decreased ability to focus thoughts, menstrual cramping, numbness, tingling, dizziness, and skin sensitivity. Many of these symptoms overlap with the symptoms of insulin resistance, metabolic syndrome, prediabetes, hypoglycemia, and type 2 diabetes. These symptoms markedly improve for many people with Metabolism B when they follow the Miracle program.

GERD (Gastric Esophageal Reflux Disease): GERD often occurs in people who have a hiatal hernia. Similar to the way that increased midline fat can affect sleep apnea, the extra fat stores around the middle can press on the stomach and cause stomach acid to backflow into the esophagus. Weight loss around the middle drastically decreases GERD's symptoms.

Glucagon: A pancreatic hormone that signals the liver to release glycogen stores and effectively stops blood glucose from dropping lower than the normal range.

Glycemic Index: Also referred to as GI, this is an index that ranks carbohydrates based on the rate at which they convert to blood glucose. The glycemic index has a scale of 0–100, with higher values given to foods that cause the most rapid rise in blood sugar. Pure glucose is the reference point, and it is given a GI of 100. For simple comparison, the foods are ranked according to their same size in weight, 50 grams. It is important to note, however, that the GI is not based on typical portion size of the food (see next entry).

Glycemic Load: GL ranks the glycemic index of foods according to the "typical" portion size of that particular food.

Glycogen: Glycogen is glucose that is formed and stored in muscle cells and in the liver. Glycogen is released from the muscles when a person exercises and is released from the liver if a person skips or delays a meal or during the sleep hours. When glycogen is released, it causes blood glucose to rise into the normal range.

Hunger: Hunger is a natural physical phenomenon. It is an unpleasant feeling experienced when one's blood sugar level begins to drop four to five hours after a meal and when the glycogen level of the liver drops below a certain threshold. The feeling associated with hunger gives us the signal to eat.

Hypertension (High Blood Pressure): Blood pressure consists of two readings: The upper reading is known as systolic and is the pressure created when your heart beats. It is considered high if it exceeds 140 mmHg. The lower reading, diastolic, is a measure of the pressure inside your blood vessels when the heart is at rest. It is considered elevated if it exceeds 90mmHg. The current recommended blood pressure goal is less than 130/80 mmHg.

Hypertension is directly related to excess weight. For those with untreated Metabolism B, continual, gradual weight gain is a matter of fact. As weight increases, so, too, does blood pressure. The permanent weight loss effected by the Metabolism Miracle will quickly help to decrease blood pressure.

Hypoglycemia: There are two types of hypoglycemia. One is caused by the excess insulin of Metabolism B, while the other is drug induced from excess glucose lowering–medication for diabetes. This temporary state of low blood sugar may come with symptoms of shaking, lightheadedness, confusion, irritability, hunger, carb cravings, cold sweats, and headache. Eating carbohydrate food immediately relieves the symptoms.

Hypoglycemia is generally classified when blood sugar dips below 70 mg/dL (3.9 mmol/L). With unchecked Metabolism B, the symptoms can occur one and a half to three hours after a meal, when the overactive pancreas pumps out excess insulin. Symptoms of hypoglycemia due to excess insulin release are a precursor to prediabetes and ultimately type 2 diabetes. A person with normal metabolism should not experience hypoglycemia. (For treatment of hypoglycemia, see chapter 12, page 190.)

Hypothyroidism: Thyroid hormones determine the speed of metabolism. When the thyroid gland can't produce enough hormone, the metabolic rate slows. Symptoms include fatigue, weakness, weight gain, or difficulty losing weight. Dry skin, constipation, muscle cramps, cold intolerance, depression, irritability, memory loss, abnormal menstrual cycles, and depressed libido can also be related to hypothyroidism. Many of the symptoms for insulin resistance, metabolic syndrome, hypoglycemia, prediabetes, and type 2 diabetes are the same. Simple blood tests are used to determine if thyroid levels are adequate and if blood sugar is in target range. Only with blood tests can one determine hypothyroidism or blood glucose abnormalities.

Injectable Insulin: Used as a medical treatment for diabetes, injectable insulin is manufactured in the laboratory using recombinant DNA.

Insulin: The hormone insulin, produced by the pancreas, helps *lower* blood glucose. Insulin acts like a key and opens the doorways into your fat and muscle cells, allowing excess glucose in your blood to move into the opened fat and muscle cells. This movement brings blood glucose back into the normal range. It also enables the glucose to be used for energy (muscle cells) or stored as fat (fat cells). Insulin is a storage hormone.

Insulin Resistance: Insulin resistance occurs when the normal amount of insulin secreted by the pancreas is not able to work effectively. When insulin does not "fit" the cell's receptors appropriately, it cannot work effectively. Eventually, the pancreas cannot keep up with the body's need for insulin, and excess glucose builds up in the bloodstream. Ironically, many people with insulin resistance have high levels of blood glucose and high levels of insulin circulating in their blood at the same time.

Liver: The liver contains a stockpile of blood sugar in the form of glycogen. Whenever you choose to skip or delay a meal and every night while you are asleep, it is your liver's release of glycogen that keeps you alive. Through the liver's intervention, the human body has the ability to "self-feed."

Metabolic Syndrome: This group of conditions increases your risk for diabetes, heart disease, and stroke. Symptoms include increased blood pressure, elevated insulin levels, excess body fat around the waist, elevated LDL cholesterol, elevated triglycerides, decreased HDL cholesterol, prediabetes, and type 2 diabetes. A major root cause of metabolic syndrome is insulin resistance.

Midline Fat Deposits: One of the hallmarks of this genetic predisposition to Metabolism B is a roll of fat around the middle. Some people also note increased "back fat." This hallmark fat deposit around the middle even occurs in otherwise thin patients.

Net Carbohydrate: The amount of carbohydrate that will eventually convert to blood glucose. Net carbohydrate is *included* in the total carbohydrate grams on a food label. Use the following formula to determine net carbs: Total carbohydrate grams - dietary fiber grams = net carbohydrate grams

Never subtract "sugar alcohol" from total carbohydrate to find a net carb, as a portion of sugar alcohol grams will convert to blood glucose.

Normal Blood Glucose Range: A person with normal carbohydrate metabolism will have blood glucose between 65 and 140 mg/dL (3.6 and 7.8 mmol/L) regardless of what he or she chooses to eat or not eat. In terms of normal blood glucose metabolism, a person can choose to fast for two days or eat a half pound of pasta with a loaf of garlic bread, and in either case, his or her blood glucose will remain in the 65–140 mg/dL range. Blood glucose is hormonally regulated by the pancreas with the help of the hormones insulin and glucagon.

Osteoarthritis: OA, a low-grade inflammation and decreased lubricating fluid in the joints, causes abnormal wearing of the protective cartilage that covers the joints. As the protection of the joints decreases, simple activities such as walking and standing become painful. Activity gradually decreases, which can compromise the functioning of muscles and ligaments. Increased body weight caused by metabolic syndrome causes osteoarthritis to be more painful and advance faster.

Osteopenia: Osteopenia occurs when bone density dips below normal. Regular exercise along with calcium and vitamin D supplementation help to alleviate the problem. If left untreated, osteopenia can lead to osteoporosis.

Osteoporosis: In this disease, bone mineral density is so compromised that an increased risk of bone fracture results. Hypothyroidism and type 2 diabetes contribute to the condition. Regular exercise, along with calcium and vitamin D supplementation, helps to prevent the condition.

Pancreas: The dual function gland/organ responsible for producing hormones that regulate blood sugar (insulin and glucagon) and digestive enzymes. Insulin and glucagon keep blood glucose in the normal range of 65–140 mg/dL (3.6–7.8 mmol/L).

Polycystic Ovarian Syndrome (PCOS): This endocrine disorder affects more than 10 percent of all women. Possibly caused by insulin resistance and the genes related to type 2 diabetes, its symptoms include irregular, few, or absent menstrual periods; depression; acne, oily skin, or dark patches of skin; infertility; hirsutism (excessive or increased body hair affecting face, chest, legs); and insulin resistance.

Sleep Apnea: In this sleep disorder, long pauses in breathing during sleep cause people to miss a number of breaths throughout the night. Lifestyle changes, such as weight loss, help arrest the loud snoring, restless sleep, and daytime sleepiness that go along with sleep apnea. Untreated Metabolism B accumulates fat around the middle, which puts pressure on the diaphragm during sleep. The Metabolism Miracle's fat-burning steps decrease midline fat and help decrease pressure on the diaphragm, thereby helping to alleviate sleep apnea.

Sleep Disturbance: Two different sleep disturbances occur with uncontrolled Metabolism B. One is the inability of the brain to relax and allow the person to fall asleep, even when the body is legitimately tired. The other disturbance occurs when a person falls asleep easily, awakens in the middle of the night, and cannot return to sleep. Both sleep disturbances seem to be caused by peaks and valleys of blood sugar during the night.

ACKNOWLEDGMENTS

Michael Scott Simon, Esq.: My heartfelt thanks for your involvement in every step of the way as *The Metabolism Miracle* progressed from my dream to a reality. Your endless energy, enthusiasm, perfectionism, tenacity, and support helped me from the first day of this project. I can never thank you enough, TB.

Andrea Somberg: My agent at the Harvey Klinger agency. Thank you for seeing the promise in the manuscript and for working to get it into the best hands.

Matthew Lore: My original publisher and editor. Your energy, intelligence, professionalism, and creativity have been greatly appreciated throughout the initial phase of this process. Thank you for taking on my life's work, recognizing the importance of "the Miracle," being open-minded through the entire process, and patiently teaching me the ropes.

Wendy Francis: Senior Editor. Thank you for taking over *The Metabolism Miracle* in the middle of the game. You have been positive, calm, collected, and professional. Thanks for all you did to make "the Miracle" a reality. Kudos to you!

Allison Cleary: My editor/writer and friend. Thank you so very much for all you put into the editing of *The Metabolism Miracle*. You are a phenomenal writer and editor with a God-given talent for making concepts come to life. You were an absolute pleasure to work with, always professional, always open, ever sharing, a consummate professional. I look forward to working with you again in future endeavors!!! Wendie Carr and Perseus Publicity Department. Thank you for the interest, professionalism, and help you channeled into publicizing the Miracle.

Cisca Schreefel, senior project editor, and Iris Bass, copy editor. Thank you for the meticulous job you did with this project. Your creativity, knowledge, and perfectionism are greatly appreciated.

Lindsey Triebel, marketing manager, and the marketing department at Da Capo Lifelong Books. Thanks for the energy, enthusiasm, and professionalism you invested in the marketing of the Miracle.

Phil Kresefski: My husband and childhood sweetheart. You've been by my side since we were children. Thank you for standing beside me in all of life's adventures. You always encourage me to be creative, trust in myself, stay positive, and work toward my dreams. Thank you for your patience and help during the countless hours involved in this process.

Diana Kresefski: My daughter and best friend. You have been a consistent source of strength, encouragement, laughs, and reality checks. You are wise beyond your years and are sure to go far in your life. Thank you for working beside me every day and keeping the Nutrition Center of Morristown (NCOM) running smoothly. I am so very proud of you.

Phillip Kresefski: My son, my heart. Thank you for your support and love. You are already an accomplished student-athlete and a wonderful, caring son. I am so very proud of you.

Ann and Bill Haduch: My parents. Your life's example motivated me to persevere, push the limits, strive for success, and above all . . . keep a positive attitude. Because of your influence, I appreciate the beauty that life has to offer.

Raymond Kresefski, Sr.: My father-in-law, the finest human being I've ever met: strong, selfless, caring, unconditionally loving. I am thankful to have had you in my life. Rest in peace.

Edward Shebol: God bless you, Grandpa. Thank you for always being there with your strength, intelligence, humor, and prayers.

(JI, DG, DF), (MN, RC, CC, TC, GS, SS): Thank you for fueling my fire to move on. Without your influence, I would never have chosen the path that led to this book.

Carmella Kresefski: Thank you for the countless hours you spent with me during the writing of this book.

My wonderful patients from the NCOM: A special thank-you to all of my patients (many of whom I count among my friends) whom I've worked with at the Nutrition Center of Morristown. Your insights, trials/tribulations, successes, and your lives are intertwined on every page of *The Metabolism Miracle*. Thank you for everything you have taught me along the way. I wish all of you all of the best.

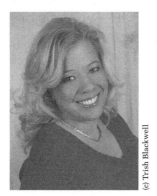

(c) Trish Blackwell

Diane Kress, **RD, CDE,** is a registered dietitian and certified diabetes educator with more than twenty-five years' experience in medical nutrition therapy. She is well known in the New York–New Jersey–Connecticut tristate area as a leading authority on innovative diet counseling. After years of practicing as a traditional nutritionist, she researched and developed the proprietary program presented in this book, specifically for those patients who could not succeed with traditional diets. *The Metabolism Miracle* has already provided over three thousand of her private practice patients with remarkable results involving permanent weight loss and decreased medications with improved blood sugar, blood pressure, cholesterol, and overall well-being.

Diane Kress's specialty areas include dietary treatment of morbid obesity, weight reduction, diabetes management and prevention, metabolic syndrome, and cardiac care nutrition. She has worked in the clinical settings of hospitals, has consulted for school systems, and currently owns and directs her own private practice, the Nutrition Center of Morristown, in Morristown, New Jersey.

Kress is a member of the American Dietetic Association, American Association of Diabetes Educators, and American Diabetes Association and has been affiliated with the Garden State Association of Diabetes Educators. She has authored articles for newspapers and is a well-known speaker at medical programs throughout New Jersey. She lives in New Jersey with her husband and two children.

Boldface page references indicate photographs. <u>Underscored</u> references indicate boxed text or charts.